"A great and timely book! Every fat conscious person should read *Anti-Fat Nutrients*."

— Ann Louise Gittleman
author of *Beyond Pritikin*

ANTI-FAT NUTRIENTS

DALLAS CLOUATRE, Ph.D.

PAX PUBLISHING • SAN FRANCISCO,CA

The writings contained in this book are provided solely for informational purposes. A physician should be consulted before embarking on any new diet, exercise or vitamin supplementation program. The nutritional substances mentioned in this book are generally regarded as safe by the Food and Drug Administration when used as recommended. However, the FDA does not recognize their use as agents for altering fat metabolism.

Pax Publishing
P.O. Box 22564
San Francisco, CA 94122

Copyright ©1997 by Dallas Clouatre, Ph.D.

ISBN 0-9614914-6-9
Library of Congress Catalog Card Number: 93-14867

Editorial Consultation: James Arden

Library of Congress Cataloging in Publication Data
Clouatre, Dallas.
Anti-Fat Nutrients: Dallas Clouatre. --2nd ed.
1. Reducing. 2. Fat-Metabolism. 3. Vitamins.
4. Dietary supplements. I. Title.
RM222.2.C52   1993   613.2'5--dc20

THIRD EDITION
First printing 1997
Six printings of previous editions.

PRINTED IN THE UNITED STATES OF AMERICA

CONTENTS

CONTENTS

CONTENTS

CONTENTS

BEYOND DIETING

This new third edition is similar in design and format to previous editions. Important updates have been made to several sections as well as the addition of new Anti-Fat Nutrients.

Until recently, "dieting" was considered to be the principle method for losing weight. At universities and nutritional research centers around the world this view is rapidly changing.

A new study by the National Institute of Health suggests that there is no evidence that caloric restriction is a good *long-term* strategy for weight loss. In fact, for some people cutting back on calories will lead to health risks.[1]

Certainly, those who significantly *over*eat can benefit from reducing their caloric intake. In general, however, calorie counting is not the solution to weight problems.

Many diets are initially effective for achieving rapid weight loss, but the weight is quickly regained once the diet is over because the pounds lost consisted primarily of water and lean muscle tissue. The result of the typical diet is that the percentage of the body's tissues made up of fats commonly is increased and the percentage made up of lean tissues which burn calories is decreased! The energy balances in the body are upset and future diets become more difficult because the body no longer responds. This is why the typical diet leads to the "yo-yo" pattern of weight loss-weight gain, with each cycle of weight gain more extreme than the previous one.

A successful weight-loss program doesn't just take off unwanted pounds, it helps you feel good and look good—permanently. This is because it includes making changes in body composition and metabolism which increase the body's ability to burn calories. These changes do not depend upon a large reduction in calories consumed, but upon modifications in the foods eaten and upon the addition of a small number of nutritional supplements to the diet. The result is a decrease in fatty tissue and an increase in the ratio of lean muscle tissue to adipose (fat) tissue in the body. Such a change is psychologically satisfying as well because lean tissue not only burns calories, but also gives women and men their shapely figures and muscle tone. In any successful weight-loss program, you should be able to judge the results by your mirror, not just your bathroom scale.

This book is divided into six chapters. The focus of these chapters is as follows:

Chapter 1 introduces new directions in the study of weight control and outlines the important contributions nutrients can make in our lives.

Chapter 2 explores nineteen key nutrititional supplements and the ways in which they facilitate weight loss.

Chapter 3 contains the Core Anti-Fat Nutrient Weight Loss Program. This section also includes nutrient programs to help reduce stress, relieve depression, and control appetite.

Chapter 4 covers the main elements of food and nutrition and offers dietary guidelines that will accelerate the weight loss process.

Chapter 5 discusses the pitfalls of dieting as a method to control weight, reveals the real causes of obesity in America, introduces the importance of our metabolic individuality and examines some of the most popular diets of this century.

Chapter 6 examines the confusion surrounding the cholesterol issue and shows how nutrients control cholesterol and help prevent heart disease.

The solution to weight management requires a multifaceted approach involving nutrition, biochemistry, psychology, exercise and lifestyle. This book provides insight into some of these factors which will enable the reader to achieve greater weight control.

Acknowledgements

The author would like to thank Dr. Jin-Bin Wu, Ph.D. in phytochemistry from Tokyo University and Professor at the College of Traditional Chinese Medicine in Taichung, Taiwan for his generous contributions to this project. The author would also like to thank Keiichi Morishita, President of The International Natural Medicine Society, for the donation of his work *The Theory of Food as The Main Factor of Cancer and Diettics*. Special thanks go to Bill Karneges of Pax Publishing for numerous suggestions for improving the structure and presentation of this material.

CHAPTER 1

Getting Lean With Nutrients

Millions of people worldwide are discovering the value which extra vitamin and other nutritional supplements can bring to their lives. For greater energy and healthier skin as well as for prolonging life and treating disease, vitamin and nutritional therapy is fast becoming the wave of the future.

Now researchers are uncovering the role certain vitamins, herbs and other nutrients can play in helping you control your weight. From nutrients which increase the amount of fat that is burned for energy to others which control sugar cravings, this book contains the latest scientific information on these "Anti-Fat Nutrients" and offers a program to help you lose weight and improve your health in a safe and effective manner.

Countless books have been written on dieting, exercise and the psychology of overeating. Certainly these factors are important, but a significant area pertaining to weight control has remained relatively unexplored, namely, the biochemistry of weight loss. *This book is unique because it offers what other approaches to weight loss cannot, a greater efficiency in fat metabolism!* This is achieved through the proper use of what we refer to as "Anti-Fat Nutrients."

It has become apparent that "dieting" (restricting calories) is not the solution to permanent weight loss. Although overeating may be the cause of weight gain in some individuals, many overweight people do not overeat. *These people are more likely the victims of inefficient fat metabolism.* These individuals need an approach which addresses the digestion, absorption, storage, and utilization of fat in the body.

Anti-Fat Nutrients are those nutritional substances which work at the biochemical level to reduce appetite and increase caloric expenditure.

Some of these nutrients interfere with fat storage or increase the use of body fat as an energy source. Others through a process called "partitioning" convince the body to use most of the calories consumed to feed lean tissues and for energy rather than to add to fat stores. The use of such Anti-Fat Nutrients has resulted in weight loss and in the increased ability to prevent new weight gain by thousands of individuals.

In just a few days after starting this program you will experience greater energy and more control over your appetite. If you have a "sweet tooth," your craving for sweets will effortlessly go away. Will power is unnecessary when your biochemistry is brought into balance. Best of all, you will be losing body fat rather than muscle tissue. Anti-Fat Nutrients encourage the burning of fat—unlike dieting, which encourages the loss of lean tissue.

The nutrients described in this book all have a variety of functions and benefits. L-Carnitine, for instance, carries fat to what are called the mitochondria in the cells, where the fat is then burned for energy. However, this nutrient not only helps you get leaner, it also helps to strengthen the heart. This illustrates one of the great strengths of nutrients: they tend to have many side benefits.

From the knowledge we have gained about the roles which these nutrients play, we have discovered how particular nutrients influence the body's decisions on when and where to metabolize (burn off) its fat deposits.

Certain nutrients are key factors in determining our body's tendency towards obesity or leanness. By choosing to include these nutrients in our diet, we gain a measure of control over our metabolism and acquire some say in how much our body gains or loses fat.

A truly effective weight control program must address the issue of fat metabolism at the biochemical level. It must take into consideration not just calories, but also the many factors which can impair fat metabolism.

Towards that end, the discussion of Anti-Fat Nutrients in this book provides a more complete understanding of how and why we gain and lose weight.

Now, let us turn to the Anti-Fat Nutrients.

CHAPTER 2

THE ANTI-FAT NUTRIENTS

#1
L-CARNITINE

Anti-Fat Nutrient	L-Carnitine.
Fat Burning Function	Shuttles fat to where it is burned for energy.
Suggested Dose	500-2000 mg in divided doses between meals.

L-CARNITINE
In Depth

What Is It?

L-carnitine is an amino acid and is also known as vitamin B . It is supplied in the diet primarily through animal muscle meats (from those of sheep and lamb in particular), and it also is manufactured in the body, mainly in the liver and the kidneys. Produced from the essential amino acid lysine, the body's synthesis of L-carnitine requires the vitamins C, B-6 and niacin, along with iron and the amino acid methionine. In humans L-carnitine is concentrated in the heart and the skeletal muscles, and also in the brain and in the sperm.

How L-Carnitine Can Help You Lose Fat

The primary role of L-carnitine in the body is as a biocatalyst. It serves to transport fatty acids across the membrane of the cell and into the mitochondria, where these fatty acids are burned for energy. It also aids in the removal of waste products from the mitochondria. (See the section later on brown fat.) L-carnitine, moreover, increases the rate of oxidation of fats in the liver, and this suggests that it plays a role in improving energy generation from this angle as well.[2] Its impact upon fat metabolism is sufficient that the *Physician's Desk Reference* has recommended dosages of 600-1200 mg. three times per day for the treatment of some forms of heart disease and for some conditions involving elevated blood lipids.

There is no scientific doubt that a cellular deficiency of carnitine can lead to symptoms such as fatigue, muscle weakness, obesity, and elevated blood lipid and triglyceride levels. Moreover, carnitine itself is very safe, so supplementation may provide insurance in cases of question. There are many anecdotal instances in which the supplement has helped to reduce excess weight, and Jeffrey Bland, Director of the Bellevue Medical Laboratory, has argued that in the proper dosages, carnitine supplementation during dieting can help to control the negative effects of ketosis (the accumulation of waste products of fat metabolism) in those who are susceptible to this problem.[3] There is also evidence that some forms of obesity may be related to a genetic propensity to produce less carnitine, and liver and kidney problems will similarly reduce the body's production since some four fifths of our carnitine total is produced internally by these organs.[4]

Finally, L-carnitine penetrates into the mitochondria themselves. It is here that most of the free radicals are generated as food is oxidized to produce energy. There is some evidence that L-carnitine serves to spare antioxidants, such as vitamin C, although the mechanism by which this is done has not yet been uncovered.

Two caveats are in order. First, some researchers argue that increasing the level of carnitine in the system does not increase the rate or the amount of fatty acids used for energy except in cases of deficiency or in cases of special disorders. The experiences of healthy athletes with supplementation have been mixed. However, the results with healthy athletes are probably not appropriate for comparisons with those of individuals suffering from excess weight or related difficulties. More importantly, current findings indicate that the mixed results came about because earlier researchers did not know what to look for and were not using the appropriate dosage levels.[5]

Second, a few authorities recommend that L-carnitine not be taken in instances of active kidney or liver disease. This caution is a matter of dispute in as much as other authorities actually suggest that supplemental carnitine aids in the treatment of some forms of kidney malfunction. However, those with active liver or kidney disease and those with diabetes or a propensity toward diabetes should follow a conservative course of action and consult their physician.

Other Benefits of L-Carnitine

—Reduces fatigue.

— Used therapeutically in the treatment of atherosclerotic heart disease.

— Increases the levels of HDL (the desirable high-density lipoprotein lipids) in the blood while decreasing the levels of tryglycerides and LDL cholesterol.

— Reduces ketone levels in the blood.

— May increase the motility and the fertility of sperm.

— May improve liver performance in cases of alcohol abuse.

— May improve some forms of kidney disease.

How Is It Available and How Should It Be Taken?

L-carnitine is available in 250 mg. capsules at most health food stores. Some companies supply 500 mg. size capsules as well. The dosage should always be taken on an empty stomach. Liquid Carnitine is also available, but some people find the glycerin base to be too sweet. Liquids tend to speed absorption, but are not necessarily as stable or as tolerable as capsules and tablets. The dosages commonly suggested for improved fat metabolism are 500 to 2000 mg. daily in separate doses. To prevent the possibility of developing a tolerance at these dosage levels, it is advisable to discontinue taking L-carnitine for one week out of each month. Only the L-form of carnitine should be taken, never the D or DL forms, which have side effects.

Those whose livers and kidneys are functioning properly can effectively increase their carnitine levels by increasing their consumption of lysine-containing foods (especially fish and the dark meat of poultry) and by adding vitamin C and the other nutrients needed for carnitine production. One study showed that adding as little as 200 mg. of vitamin C to the daily diet increased carnitine synthesis in the body. If supplemental lysine is taken, 500 mg. to 1 gram total in divided dosages taken daily before meals has been recommended. Supplementation with vitamin B5 (pantothenic acid or preferably its active coenzyme form pantethine) improves the action of Carnitine by increasing the production of Acetyl CoA in the body. Research suggests that carnitine works synergistically with coenzyme Q_{10} and pantethine. Also, supplementing with choline (20mg/kg body wight) may reduce body urinary carnitine losses as much as 75%.[6]

Recently, good results with obese subjects were achieved with a low calorie, low fat diet over an eight-week period using the following three supplements.[7]

Chromium picolinate	400 mcg.
L-carnitine	200 mg.
Fiber	20 gm.

ANTI-FAT NUTRIENT

#2
GH RELEASERS

Anti-Fat Nutrient	L-Ornithine and others.
Fat Burning Function	Mobilizes fat stores, increases muscle synthesis.
Suggested Dose	Gradual increase to 3 grams at bedtime on an empty stomach.

GROWTH HORMONE RELEASERS
In Depth

What Are They?

Growth hormone releasers are amino acids and other compounds which can stimulate the pituitary gland's secretion of growth hormone (GH). The most commonly suggested releasers are L-arginine, L-ornithine, L-tyrosine (better used as an appetite suppressant), L-tryptophan (recently banned by the FDA on questionable grounds) and L-glycine. Taken individually or in combination, these amino acids are reputed to raise the body's serum level of growth hormone. L-arginine and L-ornithine are the substances which comprise the most highly advertised night-time weight-loss products over the last few years.[8] The essential amino acid valine may prove to be more effective than either arginine and ornithine as a GH releaser when taken orally, but relatively little research has been performed to date with this amino acid.

Growth hormone is a natural hormone manufactured and stored in the pituitary gland. During our growing years, this hormone is responsible for the accelerated growth of our bones and muscles, for wound healing, for resistance to disease, and for the metabolism of fat stores. Unfortunately, the level of GH released gradually declines as we age, dropping rapidly after age 30 and becoming negligible after age 50. The pituitary does not cease producing GH, but for reasons not well understood, the aging body gradually loses its ability to release the hormone. Obese individuals also seem less able to release GH, and obesity itself can play a causative role. The goal of GH release programs is to raise the levels of GH release to those of adolescence or young adulthood.

Growth hormone is normally released one half hour into sleep, during peak exercise, and in response to fasting/food deprivation. Vitamin B-6 is necessary for GH release, and supplemental choline and vitamin B-5 also may help. Evidence even points to a role for the important antioxidant, vitamin C.

How GH Releasers Work

Growth hormone has many functions in the body. It stimulates protein production and collagen production, so it maintains and increases muscle tissue mass and it improves skin quality and the tone of the deeper layers of the dermis. More importantly for the dieter, GH causes fat stores to release fatty acids and it forces these to be burned for energy.

The release of GH is controlled by two antagonistic hormones secreted by the hypothalamus gland of the brain. As its name suggests, the growth hormone releasing hormone (GHRH) causes the pituitary gland to release GH. The other hormone, somatostatin, turns off GH release. As we age, we become more sensitive to somatostatin and its inhibitory effects upon GH release. Aging slows down other aspects of GH release as well. For instance, aging diminishes the production of the neurotransmitter acetylcholine, and it thereby again reduces the responsiveness to GHRH.

Furthermore, changes in insulin response are heavily implicated in the decline in responsiveness to GHRH and in the increase in sensitivity to somatostatin. GH release is usually triggered by low blood sugar levels, whereas somatostatin release is triggered by high blood sugar levels. Anything which upsets the insulin mechanism of the body therefore upsets GH release. Obesity, diets based upon simple carbohydrates and, diets lacking in chromium and other insulin-potentiating nutrients all will negatively affect GH release.[9]

Not all of the factors which cause declines in GH can be influenced, but certainly some can. The question is "How much?" The usual supplements employed are L-arginine and L-ornithine, either alone or in combination. Most of the successful research results involved the injection of these amino acids, not their ingestion by mouth. Injection certainly produced dramatic results, but human tests with oral supplements often have shown only slight effects.[10] However, recent medical studies on burn and surgical patients have indicated that the alpha-ketoglutarate form of ornithine successfully maintains muscle mass and protein synthesis during severe trauma, i.e., the effects of GH release.[11] GABA (gamma amino butyric acid) is another special amino acid which appears to successfully cause the release of GH.[12]

Those suffering from seriously excessive weight gain tend not to respond well to GH releasers. Moreover, responsiveness to GH releasers declines in everyone after the age of 30. The consensus is that we continue to produce adequate levels of GH, but that for some reason this GH is not as readily released into the blood stream as during our younger years.

Other Benefits of GH Releasers

L-Arginine
- Stimulates the immune system.
- Promotes wound healing.
- Blocks the formation of tumors.
- Helps to regenerate the liver.
- Increases spermatogenesis.

L-Ornithine
- Stimulates the immune system.
- Promotes wound healing.
- Scavenges free radicals.
- Helps to regenerate the liver.

(Arginine and ornithine consumption in excess may activate arthritic symptoms and likewise activate a previously dormant herpes virus. Since these amino acids must exist in a balance with the essential amino acid lysine in the body, excessive consumption of their pure forms may create a lysine deficiency.)

L-Tyrosine
- Helps to control depression/anxiety.
- Acts as an appetite suppressant.
- Acts as a mild antioxidant.
- Increases the production of melanin.
- Is a precursor to a thyroid hormone, as is L-phenylalanine.

L-Glycine
- Effective for hyperacidity (often used as an antacid).
- Used as a food additive for its sweet taste.
- An important component of the body's antioxidant enzyme glutathione peroxidase.
- May promote healing, especially when taken with arginine or ornithine.

GABA   -   Lowers blood pressure and encourages sleep.
- Considered an anti-stress, anti-anxiety nutrient

How Are They Available and How Should They Be Taken?

The quantity of amino acids in formulas varies with the source, as does the price. The usual procedure is to gradually increase the dosage over several days until a maximal dosage has been reached. Results are obtained by taking the amino acids with adequate amounts of water on an empty stomach at bedtime, that is, 2 to 4 hours after meals. Sugars and refined carbohydrates should not be consumed in the meals eaten either before or after taking GH releasers. Most amino acids can also be taken upon arising and about 1 hour before meals. GABA, however, causes relaxation and should usually only be taken at night.

More is not necessarily better. Large amounts of pure amino acids will cause diarrhea, upset the stomach, and interfere with sleep. Some authorities suggest that it is best to combine one gram of L-arginine with one gram of L-ornithine at bedtime. Others suggest higher dosages, perhaps 5-6 grams. GABA is taken in dosages of only 1-2 grams. L-Glycine again requires much higher dosages and should be taken according to the manufacturer's instructions. Use of GH releasers should always be cycled; the use of pure amino acids should be discontinued for at least one week per month.

For convenience and effectiveness, many companies now sell formulas which already combine two or more GH-releasing amino acids, usually arginine/ornithine. Other formulas contain L-carnitine (see the discussion of this nutrient given earlier). The combination of L-arginine pyroglutamate/lysine may be more effective than is L-arginine alone.

Recent   research has added new GH releasers to the list of effective supplements. As little as 2 grams of the amino acid L-glutamine may improve GH release. Between 8 and 10 grams of arginine aspartate has been shown to normalize GH release patterns in aging subjects to those of younger adults. (Fourth Annual Anti-Aging Conference, Las Vegas, 1996.)

Since vitamin B-6 is necessary for the maximum effectiveness of these amino acids, it is added to some of their formulations. Other nutrients important for GH release include acetylcholine precursors, such as choline (or the more concentrated phosphatidyl choline) and vitamin B-5 (pantothenic acid) which likewise can be purchased from these companies. Recommendations for the latter are usually 3 grams of choline and 1 gram of B-5 taken in divided doses.

GABA is commonly counterfeited, so it should be purchased only from reputable firms. The alpha-ketoglutarate form of ornithine is only now becoming available, so it, too, should be purchased only after careful selection.

CAUTIONS

Those who are diabetic or borderline diabetic should avoid taking GH releasers. Those who are in doubt should consult their physicians. Supplemental chromium and/or vanadyl sulfate may be wise for anyone taking these amino acids on a regular basis. Likewise, too much arginine/ornithine will imbalance their proper ratio to the amino acid lysine in the body. This imbalance has been implicated in aggravating a prexisting herpes condition in sensitive individuals and it may negatively affect other lysine-dependent reactions.

#3

GLA

Anti-Fat Nutrient	GLA (Gamma-Linolenic Acid)
Fat Burning Function	Increases brown fat activity which burns fat for energy.
Suggested Dose	2-8 500 mg capsules in divided doses with meals.

GLA (Gamma-Linolenic Acid) AND
THE ESSENTIAL FATTY ACIDS
In Depth

What Is It?

Gamma-linolenic acid (GLA) is a fatty acid nutrient. Under ideal circumstances it is made in the body from the conversion of linoleic acid, one of the two essential fatty acids (EFA's). GLA technically is an Omega-6 fatty acid. It serves as a precursor to a family of hormone-like substances or "activated fatty acids" known as prostaglandins (PG), in particular the series called PGE-1, meaning the prostaglandin family "E" derived from GLA. The PGE-1 family is involved in anti-inflammatory, anti-spasm, anti-infection and similar actions in the body, including reducing the "stickiness" of the blood.

A second family of prostaglandins (PGE-2) is made from linoleic acid through an intermediate step creating arachidonic acid and also directly from the arachidonic acid readily found in the American diet. This PGE-2 series activates aspects of the immune and other systems, but in excess it leads to inflammation, menstrual cramps, asthma, heart disease and many other problems, including in some cases obesity. Among its other duties, the PGE-1 family serves to control or to turn off the PGE-2 family.

Many factors can prevent the conversion of linoleic acid to GLA and from there to PGE-1. These factors include deficiencies of the vitamins B-3, B-6, C, and biotin and of the minerals magnesium and zinc. Too much alcohol, too much saturated fat, the consumption of hydrogenated and heat-damaged fats and many other dietary factors are involved. Moreover, many people (especially those who tend to put on weight) have difficulty in transforming linoleic acid into GLA simply because they naturally produce relatively little of the enzyme needed for this transformation.[13]

How GLA Can Help You Lose Fat

A study conducted in 1979 illustrates the effectiveness of GLA as a nutrient promoting weight loss. In this study, thirty-eight individuals took GLA in the form of evening primrose oil for eight weeks. Of the subjects who were more than 10% above their ideal weights, half lost an average of 9 pounds while taking four capsules per day. Only five individuals in the group showed no weight change, and the four subjects who took eight capsules per day averaged a weight loss of 23 pounds. One explanation of the effectiveness of GLA is that it appears to increase the level of brown fat NA/K ATPase activity. Brown fat, as pointed out in Chapter 5, readily burns fat stores for energy, and this specific enzyme (NA/K ATPase) controls the rate of metabolism.[14]

GLA and similarly active products are available in various forms, but it should be emphasized that essential fatty acids are foods, and the best approach is to correct the diet even if you plan to supplement. Many factors in the diet impede the absorption of EFA's. The most important of these factors are the consumption of refined and overheated vegetable oils, the presence in the diet of margarines and other sources of hydrogenated oils with their *trans*-fatty acids which produce negative effects in the body (no, margarine is not good for you), and the consumption of too much saturated fat. Natural fats from unprocessed foods are almost entirely *cis*-fatty acids, which are of benefit to the body, and only rarely *trans*-fatty acids.

Frying with *any* polyunsaturated oil, such as peanut or cottonseed oil, damages that oil and impedes the absorption of EFA's contained both in those oils and in the foods cooked in them. Although it has a relatively low smoking point, olive oil, which is mostly monosaturated, is probably the best choice as an oil for frying. Frying with highly unsaturated oils is so unhealthful that even the much maligned animal fats may be preferable for this task to, say, safflower, corn, or other such oils. Trans-fatty acids have long been known to adversely affect the immune system, to increase free radical production, to produce abnormal sperm, to lower testosterone levels, and to impair the processing of insulin.[15]

Direct sources of GLA are expensive and difficult to keep fresh, although there are some excellent sources available. Your body can manufacture its own GLA from cis-linoleic acid, which can be found in unrefined, *cold-pressed* polyunsaturated vegetable oils. (These oils must be *cold-pressed* only. If they are not specifically labeled as such, they should be avoided)

For those who are over their ideal weights, it may be best to assume that the body's ability to create GLA may be impaired. Thus sources of pure GLA may be necessary. An alternative to supplementation with GLA is to supply the very important Omega-3 essential fatty acid known as alpha-linolenic acid (LNA). This fatty acid can be used to create the PGE-3 family of prostaglandins, and the PGE-3's can perform most of the roles of the PGE-1's. Fish oils provide the precursors to PGE-3, but these are expensive. Good plant sources are rare, but they do exist and might be tried. The richest plant source of LNA is fresh flax seed oil. (Flax seed oil always should be taken with a small amount of vitamin B-6, and it is best utilized when eaten with a bit of sulphur-containing protein, such as low-fat cottage cheese.)

More commonly available plant sources of LNA are pumpkin seed oil (15%), soy oil (9%) and walnut oil (5%). Again, .hese should be cold pressed and protected from heat and light. Fresh, raw pumpkin seeds and walnuts can be used in place of the oils. A tablespoonful of one of these cold-pressed, unrefined oils twice a day should be sufficient. The diet should be supplemented with at least 50 I.U.'s of vitamin E along with the oils to protect these fatty acids from oxidation within the body.

Other Benefits of GLA and LNA[16]

— GLA is noted for its usefulness in relieving premenstrual syndrome. (PMS)

— GLA has important anti-inflammatory properties.

— GLA helps to control rheumatoid arthritis. Evidence suggests that LNA may also work to control arthritis and other similar degenerative conditions

— Both GLA and LNA have proved effective against cancer cells in vitro, and they are used abroad in some human cancer treatments.

— Both combat heart disease by lowering blood viscosity and by reducing LDL levels. Both GLA and LNA decrease blood platelet "stickiness."

— Both combat high blood pressure.

— Both have shown usefulness in combatting acne, eczema and other skin problems.

— GLA and LNA can help prostate gland problems.

— LNA has been shown to act as a substrate for the activities of various B vitamins. A deficiency of Omega-3 fatty acids is implicated as a basic cause of major mental illnesses, and the PGE-3 family plays a role in regulating parts of the nervous system throughout the body.

— Both GLA and LNA play roles in improving immune response.

— GLA has been shown to have benefits in cases of diabetic neuropathy (nerve damage). Over the course of a year, a large dose of GLA (480 mg. daily), improved nerve status in 13 out of 16 measures in a controlled study.

How Is It Available and How Should It Be Taken?

GLA appears to be more important for improving weight control than is LNA. It is found in significant amounts in human mother's milk, in the seed oil of the evening primrose plant, borage oil, and black currant seed oil. Doses from 90 mg to as much as 400 mg of GLA have proven effective. This is the amount of GLA found in 2-8 500 mg capsules of Evening Primrose Seed Oil. Some individuals may find that they receive benefits only at the higher dosage range. GLA is often more effective when taken in conjunction with vitamin B-6 and d-alpha-tocopherol (vitamin E).

GLA has been reported to give rise to occasional mild acne. In the experience of one clinical bariatrician, large doses given to improve weight loss also may lead to increased susceptibility to bruising in a small number of individuals. GLA is an unsaturated oil, and it therefore needs protection against oxidation and free radical damage. Concurrent daily usage of vitamin E (400 to 800 IU) and grape seed extract polyphenols (100 to 200 mg.) is suggested. Fish oils may also prove helpful. These nutrients help to prevent GLA from being transformed into arachidonic acid and the "bad" prostaglandins.

ANTI-FAT NUTRIENT

#4
CHROMIUM

Anti-Fat Nutrient	Chromium,Vanadyl Sulfate.
Fat Burning Function	Cuts sugar cravings, reduces fat storage.
Suggested Dose	Chromium 200-600 mcg. Vanadyl Sulfate 5-15 mg.

CHROMIUM, VANADYL SULFATE
AND OTHER INSULIN POTENTIATORS
In Depth

What Are They and How Do They Work?

As you will see in Chapter 5, problems in carbohydrate metabolism play a large causative role in the American tendency to put on excess weight. One of the primary substances involved in fat storage is the hormone insulin, so it is reasonable to presume that foods and nutrients which make insulin more effective and which mimic insulin's actions in the body might aid in controlling appetite and weight gain. An enormous amount of scientific attention is now being directed toward a number of micro-nutrients which appear to perform just these functions. Among these are the trace minerals chromium and vanadium, the Ayur-vedic herb *Gymnema sylvestre* and some cooking herbs and spices, including bay leaves, "apple pie spice" (allspice), cinnamon, cloves and tumeric. The mechanisms by which these work vary.[17] These different insulin potentiators are taken up in the following order: chromium, vanadium and then *Gymnema sylvestre*.

Chromium has been the subject of the most study because it was discovered in 1957 to be central to a substance known as glucose tolerance factor (GTF). One form of chromium, the mineral in its trivalent state combined with niacin and the amino acids glycine, cysteine and glutamic acid, makes up GTF. Unfortunately, no one has yet learned how to manufacture or extract GTF, and chromium itself is difficult for the body to manipulate into its biologically active form.[18]

Chromium as part of GTF is thought to improve the absorption of glucose into the cells, making it more useful for energy. Since the GTF also potentiates (makes insulin more effective) the effects of insulin, less insulin is needed and blood sugar levels are stabilized. This means that energy levels also are stabilized and the extreme fluctuations of hunger associated with hypoglycemia are avoided. The usefulness to the dieter and to those with diabetic tendencies is obvious. Just as important, however, is the fact that chromium has been shown to help decrease unwanted blood lipid levels, both of LDL cholesterol and of triglycerides, while actually raising the levels of the desirable HDL fraction of the blood.[19] Many of the actions given below for vanadium apply alike to chromium and other insulin potentiators, so, with important exceptions, these substances are interchangeable.

The American diet is notoriously deficient in chromium, and it is commonly estimated that as many as 90% of all Americans are marginally deficient in chromium or worse. We certainly suffer in comparison with parts of the world in which diabetes and heart disease remain rare. Tissue levels of chromium are five times higher in most parts of Asia than in the U.S.[20] Similar low tissue levels are true of Americans tested for many other important minerals, and two likely causes are our farming methods and our processing and refining of many foods.

Current interest in the trace mineral vanadium dates to 1985 when an article in the prestigious journal *Science* indicated that vanadium controlled diabetes in laboratory animals.[21] This data created excitment because it showed that vanadium is effective when taken by mouth, whereas insulin must be injected to be effective. Other studies quickly confirmed these results, and it is now known that vanadium plays an important role not only in controlling blood sugar levels, but also, as is true of chromium, in preventing the development of excessive levels of LDL cholesterol and triglycerides.[22] Further evidence exists to the effect that vanadium assists in the development of the bones and teeth.

These impressive recent findings actually constitute a rediscovery of the uses of vanadium. In France vanadium was already a medically recommended treatment for diabetes and some forms of fatigue in the late 19th Century. In the English-speaking world, the 1932 edition of *Dorland's Medical Dictionary* listed vanadium as a treatment for diabetes and neurasthenia; with the addition of selenium, it was also suggested as a treatment for cancer. In the 1958 edition of *Dorland's*, atherosclerosis (hardening of the arteries) was added to the illnesses for which vanadium was recommended. Vanadium therefore has a track record of usage with human beings, not just with laboratory animals.

Although not as successful as injected insulin for the treatment of extreme cases of diabetes, which is the reason that it originally disappeared from medical usage, vanadium in the form of vanadyl sulfate (its biologically active form) can mimic many of the activities of insulin. In this respect vanadyl sulfate is even more impressive than is chromium. Chromium potentiates the body's insulin, but the vanadyl form of vanadium itself is biologically active even in the absence of insulin. It significantly increases liver glycogen (stored glucose) and it improves the uptake of glucose by muscle tissues. These actions help to spare lean tissue during dieting and to improve athletic performance by lessening fatigue and by reducing the breakdown of muscle protein for energy. Vanadyl sulfate thus possesses anti-catabolic properties. Nevertheless, it also acts to inhibit the storage of excess calories from carbohydrates as fat, apparently by stabilizing the body's production of insulin. These properties, again, are useful for controlling weight gain and for improving athletic performance.

The herb *Gymnema sylvestre* has been used in Indian/ Ayurvedic medicine for two millennia to control problems in carbohydrate metabolism. Animal studies have confirmed that the herb does indeed reduce blood sugar levels.[23] Other studies demonstrate that gymnema extracts increase the functions of the liver and the pancreas, areas which, as will be shown in Chapter 5, tend to have weakened functions in those who are overweight. Another factor of significance to dieters is the fact that Gymnema appears to reduce cravings for sweet foods, and it does this by affecting the taste receptors.[24] As with chromium and vanadium, this insulin potentiator appears to normalize blood lipid levels and to lower insulin requirements. However, unlike the two micronutrients, *Gymnema sylvestre* may work by repairing and/ or regenerating the insulin-producing cells of the pancreas![25]

Benefits of Insulin Potentiators

— They control blood sugar levels, and thereby affect energy levels and hunger spikes.

— They help to normalize fat storage and improve the utilization of fat for energy.

— They may help to increase lean tissue in the body and to "build muscles" in those who actively train with weights.

— They may help to prevent and to control diabetes.

— Chromium and vanadium lower blood lipid levels, and chromium may raise the level of HDL, which is desirable.[26]

— Chromium and vanadium may strengthen the immune system.

— Vanadium plays a role in the laying down of calcium in the bones and teeth.

How Are They Available and How Should They Be Taken?

Chromium is not well absorbed by the body, and there is presently enormous controversy as to which form of chromium supplement is best assimilated. Most of the research showing significant effects has been done with the picolinate or polynicotinate (ChromeMate) forms, and the consensus seems now to be that of the least expensive forms available, these may be the best. Both chromium picolinate and polynicotinate are sold by most of the leading vitamin companies. Since absorption is poor for almost any form, 200 mcg. is likely a safe long term dosage for any individual. Therapeutic dosages may be as much as 1,000 mcg. per day, although such a high intake probably should not continue for more than a few months without an interval. *Only the trivalent form of chromium should be taken.*

There is no currently accepted Recommended Daily Allowance (RDA) for vanadium, although it is recognized that a deficiency of this trace mineral is detrimental to both animal and human health. The average diet provides roughly 2 mg. of the elemental form per day from fats and vegetable oils, and in some parts of the world, particularly in areas of South America, diets provide 10-15 mg. of elemental vanadium per day, which is quite high. Absorption is usually only about 5-10% of that ingested and the unused amount is readily excreted. The recommended supplemental dosage of vanadyl sulfate is 1-2 mg. per day, and more for special purposes. Some studies have used 22.5 mg. of vanadyl sulfate per day for 16 months without toxic effects, but others report that this amount is actually in excess of what can be absorbed, and that no further benefits can be expected in dosages over 15 mg. of vanadyl sulfate per day, with the exception of diabetics under medical supervision. In other words, there is no consensus on effective dosage levels. The vanadate forms of vanadium should not be taken as supplements.[27] A new form of vanadium, bis(maltolato)oxovanadium(IV), has recently been developed which is both more potent and even safer than is vanadyl sulfate.

Gymnema sylvestre is sometimes included in diet formulas for its effect upon the perception of sweetness. However, this is of somewhat questionable benefit to most individuals. The more appropriate use of the herb is for its insulin-potentiating effects and its effects upon the liver and pancreas. For these purposes, the whole herb should probably be used. The Indian common name for the plant is Shardunika.

Some of the most potent regulators of insulin are also the most pleasant to use. Good quality cinnamon, although not inexpensive, is very useful in this regard, as are allspice, cloves and tumeric (curcumin). Tumeric has the added advantage of being a liver detoxifier and an anti-inflammatory. Bay leaves, although too strong to use in great quantity, improve digestion of legumes and fats and have been used since ancient times for their healthful properties.

CAUTION

There is a clinically recognized form of depression which is treated with a low-vanadium diet. This syndrome is genetic and not vanadium-induced, but those being treated for depression should consult their physician before adding vanadium to their diets. Those taking MAO inhibitors should not take vanadium supplements. Corrections of elevated blood glucose levels may also leave one *temporarily* tired. This may result from the use of insulin potentiators and mimics.

Some insulin resistant individuals may find the Gymnema sylvestre increases insulin levels too much, which can elevate blood pressure in rare cases. These individuals should employ other insulin potentiators to improve their insulin sensitivity.

#5
NATURAL APPETITE SUPPRESSANTS

Anti-Fat Nutrient	L-Tyrosine and others.
Fat Burning Function	Stimulates the release of CCK, which controls appetite.
Suggested Dose	250-1000 mg divided doses on an empty stomach with water.

NATURAL APPETITE SUPPRESSANTS (ANORECTICS)
In Depth

What Are They and How Do They Work?

There are a number of natural appetite suppressants available both as supplements and through food sources. Foods which work to reduce hunger include fiber (see the separate Fiber section below) and the blue-green algae called spirulina. Supplements which act as anorectics, that is, appetite suppressants, include the amino acids L-phenylalanine and L-tyrosine. (Do not use the D- or DL- forms for this purpose.) A powerful anorectic herb known to Arabic folk medicine and used in Europe for weight loss is wall germander (Teucrium polium). The thermogenic aids described later in this book also can act as appetite suppressants. These include caffeine and the herb Ma Huang. Similarly, natural lipogenesis inhibitors (items which inhibit fat storage, for which see the special Lipogenesis Inhibitors section later in this book) generally double as anorectics. Not yet available or just coming onto the market are pharmaceutical anorectics which work by preventing the storage of calories as fat.

It is sometimes suggested that the amino acid L-glutamine (not glutamic acid) can help to control sugar and alcohol cravings. The mechanism is unclear, although there is experimental support for the notion that an appetite control center in the brain is involved.[28]

Glutamine in an animal test caused mice to lose 10% of their body weight, reduced blood sugar levels 50% and reduced insulin levels 30%, even when the animals were fed a high fat diet (45%). In a second experiment using a high fat diet, the unsupplemented animals gained 15% in weight, yet the glutamine group gained no weight over a two month period.[29]

The hormone Cholecystokinin (CCK) was also available as an anorectic until 1985. CCK is an important key to appetite control. Since it plays a large part in the effectiveness of many of the other anorectics, it deserves some introduction. CCK is a hormone released from the hypothalamus, a section of the cerebral cortex of the brain. It is also released by the small intestine to stimulate digestion.[30] Significantly, it is one of the hormones which signals to us that we have eaten enough. (Serotonin, produced from the amino acid L-tryptophan, is another neurotransmitter which is implicated in signaling satiety.) Experiments have shown conclusively that injections of CCK into the proper area of the brain will prevent even starving rats from eating, whereas surgical damage to the hypothalamus to prevent the reception of the CCK stimulus will cause rats to eat themselves to death. Therefore, there is no doubt that the hormone is important in appetite control.

A number of immitations of CCK are still being sold, but the real item is no longer available. CCK was considered a nutritional supplement until overzealous manufacturers made claims not yet validated according to FDA regulations. These claims to drug-like effects caused the FDA to pull all CCK from stores and prevent its future sale until further clinical tests have been conducted. Considering the fact that CCK is a naturally-occurring substance and therefore unpatentable, it is highly unlikely that any company will ever put up the huge sums of money necessary to gain FDA approval. In this particular instance this may be a good thing in as much as taking any hormone requires supervision.

Safe and effective ways of stimulating the brain to release its own CCK remain available using the related amino acids L-phenylalanine and L-tyrosine, which can still be purchased. L-phenylalanine is an essential amino acid. Through a series of biochemical reactions, L-phenylalanine is easily converted by the body to L-tyrosine. In turn, L-tyrosine is a precursor to a number of neurotransmitters and hormones, such as adrenaline (norepinephrine), dopamine and thyroid hormones. This means that L-tyrosine is a precursor to important stimulants to the metabolism (including thermogenesis) and to the nervous system. L-tyrosine is a primary precursor to CCK and it also has a weak antioxidant effect.

L-phenylalanine, the natural form of the amino acid, is recognized by the FDA as a food. As an amino acid, it is available through foods which have significant protein components, especially meats, poultry and nuts. The presence of L-phenylalanine may be one of the routes by which high-protein diets serve to alleviate hunger in dieters. A number of special items, such as spirulina, combine this essential amino acid with a variety of other benefits.

Spirulina has been used as a food by Central American and African tribes for centuries. It is now farmed and cultivated on a large scale in California, Mexico, Japan and elsewhere. It is sold around the world as a natural food supplement rich in nutrients. Over the last several years it has been used by many people as an effective aid to weight loss. Spirulina contains substantial amounts of complete protein, essential fatty acids, vitamins and minerals while being nevertheless low in calories. It is known experimentally that concentrated complete foods tend to reduce the appetite and partition energy into the body's lean tissues.[31]

Other Benefits of
L-Phenylalanine and L-Tyrosine[32]

— When taken over a period of time, i.e., two weeks or more, both L-phenylalanine and L-tyrosine may help to control depression and anxiety.

— Both amino acids enhance learning, alertness and memory.

— Phenylalanine in its "D" and "DL" forms is often effective for the control of chronic pain as these forms interfere with the degradation of endorphins (the body's own natural pain-killers). These forms are less useful for appetite control.

— Phenyalanine/tyrosine use is sometimes associated with enhanced sex drive.

— L-Tyrosine is a minor growth hormone (GH) stimulant.

— L-Tyrosine is a precursor to thyroid hormones and may help correct mild hypothyroidism.

How Are They Available and How Should
They Be Taken?

L-glutamine is available in many health food stores and should be taken on an empty stomach in 500 mg to 4 gram dosages.

The anorectic herb wall germander has been used in Europe but, it is not commonly available in the United States and there are some questions now of liver toxicity if a related species of the herb is used. Much more accessible are thermogenic herbs which also serve to reduce the appetite such as green tea, kola nut, gurana and ephedrine-containing plants.

Since spirulina is a true food, it is quite safe and can be used like any other food. For dieting, however, best results come from taking this supplement either with breakfast or instead of breakfast, and then perhaps an hour before each of the other meals. Instructions come with the product, which also can now be purchased in tablet form, but which usually is found as a powder. At the start a single dose might be one half teaspoon in a glass of water, and gradually increased to a full teaspoon taken two or three times a day. Also be aware that there are very large differences in quality between various brands of spirulina. The top grades can be quite expensive. Some cheaper grades of spirulina have undesirable bacterial counts, so it pays to find out about the quality of the product you are purchasing.

Both L-phenylalanine and L-tyrosine are available in 500 mg. capsules, and the normal dosage is one or two capsules on an empty stomach. Many individuals can tolerate only smaller dosages at the start (see cautions below) so it is wise to begin with perhaps 250 mg. or less and then increase the dosage. Since the body stores some of these amino acids, after a period of time it may be necessary to reverse this procedure and to reduce the dosage of these amino acids. L-tyrosine is the faster acting of the two (the body produces L-tyrosine from L-phenylalanine after several hours) and it is commonly taken either before meals for better absorption, or in the evening at bedtime a few hours after the last meal. Take these amino acids in the morning if your sleep is disturbed. L-tyrosine, but not L-phenylalanine, has been shown to markedly improve the appetite suppression found with ephedrine/Ma huang.

Both L-phenylalanine and L-tyrosine require the presence of the vitamins C and B-6 for conversion into several brain neurotransmitters. Therefore, it is important to supplement your diet with these vitamins for best results.

CAUTIONS

Both L-phenylalanine and L-tyrosine can cause headaches, irritability, restlessness and insomnia in sensitive individuals or at excessive dosages. Both can raise blood pressure, and they should not be used in conjunction with phenylpropanolamine (a common over-the-counter diet aid). They should never be used in conjunction with MAO inhibitor anti-depressant drugs or in the presence of pre-existing pigmented malignant melanomas (a specific skin cancer). If in doubt about the suitability of these products for your individual condition, always take the most conservative course and consult your physician or other licensed health professional.

Since L-phenylalanine and especially L-tyrosine supply a substrate for the production of thyroid and adrenal hormones, they should be used with a bit of caution and in smaller quanti ies if taken in conjunction with thyroid and adrenal activators, such as ephedrine. Nevertheless, supplementation with L-tyrosine may help avoid the thyroid and adrenal exhaustion which is encouraged by the excessive and sustained consumption of caffeine and ephedrine, two items which are common in diet products which work primarily by increasing thermogenesis.

Artificial Appetite Suppressants

Natural anorectics are safe and effective for most individuals. Over-the-counter appetite suppressants, or diet pills, contain various artificial chemical substances. Unlike the amino acid L-phenylalanine, which contributes to the production of the brain fuel norepinephrine (NE), the artificial phenylpropanolamine will, in about two weeks, deplete the brain reserve of NE. This reduction of NE produces a number of undesirable side effects including fatigue, depression and other negative behavioral changes. Other synthetic appetite suppressants include the drugs phentermine and fenfluramine. These, too, have serious side effects.

Dexfenfluramine, a more potent form of fenfluramine marketed as Redux, has recently become a focus of medical concern because studies suggest that it significantly increases the risk of pulmonary hypertension, a rare but often fatal lung disorder. Fenfluramine and its derivatives also are implicated. Use for a period of 3 months or more increases the risk of pulmonary hypertension by 30 times.[33] There also have been reports that the use of dexfenfluramine in amounts only slightly above those commonly prescribed can lead to a radical reduction in the body's production of serotonin and even to the destruction of the cells which synthesize serotonin.

A number of brain chemicals have recently been uncovered which suppress the appetite: Leptin, glucagon-like peptide 1 (GLP-1) and, most recently discovered, the hormone urocortin. The primary site of action is the hypothalamus. Thus far, these hormones have been shown to work only via injection. Drug versions of any of them are years away.

#6
NATURAL DIGESTIVE AIDS

Anti-Fat Nutrient	Bromelain and others.
Fat Burning Function	Improve digestion of protein, carbohydrates and fats.
Suggested Dose	250-500 mg with meals.

DIGESTIVE AIDS
(Pancreatin, Bromelain, Papain, etc.)
In Depth

What Are They?

From the moment food enters the mouth, it is attacked by a variety of digestive enzymes. Enzymes are proteins which serve as catalysts for the breakdown of food components. Saliva contains *amylase* which begins the digestion of starches. The hydrochloric acid and the enzyme called *pepsin* found in the stomach digest proteins. The organ called the pancreas not only provides insulin to control blood sugar levels, but it also produces amylase to split starches into more simple sugars, other proteases (protein digesting enzymes) to further break down proteins, and *lipase* to digest fats. The liver, the gall bladder and the intestinal wall itself supply yet other digestive enzymes. The rather complex mixture of digestive elements secreted by the pancreas is commonly lumped under the single heading of *pancreatin,* which is the defatted and dried powder of raw pancreas enzymes.

A number of plant, yeast, fungal and bacterial substances can serve to improve the digestion of various components of the diet.

Bromelain, which is found in raw pineapple, and papain, which comes from papaya, are powerful protein digesting substances. The culture of *Aspergillus* (a fungus) is used similarly as the source of many active enzymes, including forms of protease, amylase, lipase, cellulase and lactase.

It should be noted that many whose digestive systems are underactive may have acquired *Candida albicans* (yeast) infections or otherwise lack the proper intestinal flora. Yeast infections are difficult to prove, but they are suspected in many cases of unexplained fatigue, water retention, weight gain, immune suppression and allergies. A number of products attempt to correct these conditions by killing the offending yeast and by supplementing the normal intestinal flora with bacteria which are known to be found in the healthy gastrointestinal tract. See the discussion "Other Digestive Issues" which concludes this section.

How They Help With Weight Loss

Since many diet products claim to work by interfering with the digestion or absorption of fats, it may seem strange that digestive aids can help one to lose weight. However, evidence points in this direction. In animal experiments, supplementation with pancreatin both reduced food intake and led to weight loss.[32] Why this should be the case is not entirely clear. Sometimes weight gain is triggered as a response to the body's perceived lack of calories or nutrients. In such instances the weight gain may be reversed following the improved digestion which comes with the use of pancreatin or following the use of nutrient-rich foods such as spirulina. In Chapter 5, the role of nutrition in shunting calories into the lean tissues and into activity will be discussed as an aspect of "partitioning." No matter what one's weight, impaired digestion, malabsorption and nutritional deficiencies will lead to ill health. In those who are overweight, the symptoms will be disproportionately those of lowered thyroid activity, sluggishness, fluid retention, inflammation and the like.

Bromelain is more narrow in its effects than is pancreatin; it is primarily involved in the digestion of protein. For best results it should be combined with pancreatin and bile. Papain, which is derived from the unripe papaya, not only digests protein, but wheat gluten as well. This is quite a bonus, for difficulty in digesting gluten is quite common.

Animal sources of digestive aids tend to be stronger and more broad-spectrum than plant and bacterial sources, with pork-derived pancreatin being much stronger than that from oxen.

Other Benefits of Digestive Aids[34]

— Pancreatin and bromelain have been shown to improve the body's response to inflammation and swelling, and therefore to be useful for diseases such as rheumatoid arthritis. Used in conjunction, bromelain improves the absorption of the pancreatin.

— Proteolytic (protein-digesting) enzymes help prevent and remove fibrin clots in blood and lymph vessels.

— Proteases improve the body's ability to remove circulating immune complexes (by-products of immune system activities) from the blood and thus protect the kidneys and improve immune responses while reducing autoimmune reactions.

— Pancreatin and other protein-digesting enzymes, by preventing undigested protein from reaching the small intestine, may serve to reduce allergies, food sensitivities and a host of other reactions to foreign proteins reaching the blood stream.

— Bromelain may block the production of the prostaglandins which make the blood "sticky."

— Bromelain and other proteolytic enzymes improve the body's ability to turn over the protein content of the tissues, and thus they help in the healing of soft tissue injuries such as those often encountered in sports.

— Bromelain may improve the absorption of antibiotics, antioxidants and other compounds into the tissues.[35]

How Are They Available and How Should They Be Taken?

Pancreatin is sold in terms of its activity or strength, not its weight. If the pancreatin is listed as 4X USP, for instance, the dosage might be 2-4 tablets with meals; at 8X or 10X the dosage would be one or two tablets. Another unit used is NF or Natural Formulary, which is of a similar potency to the U.S.P.(U.S. Pharmacopeia). Since many standards are used, there is some confusion over equivalencies among products. Pancreatin, bromelain and papain are often combined with betain HCl (hydrochloric acid) to improve digestion in the stomach. Formulas may mix a number of enzymes together, such as mixing amylase, protease, lipase and cellulase together, or adding these to a formula based upon pancreatin. Always start with a conservative dosage, work up to a satisfactory amount, and cut back the dosage as your digestive ability improves.

Bromelain and papain are sold by weight (mg.) and by potencies. The common units of activity are MCU (milk clotting units) and GDU (gelatin digesting units). For a potency of 2000 GDU, you would use 250 to 500 mg. of bromelain with meals, or 500 to 1000 mg. of papain. Many studies recommend 2000 to 4000 mg. of bromelain a day! For inflammation and other such special uses, these two enzymes are taken between meals rather than with. However, those with ulcers or similar gastrointestinal problems should consult their doctors before trying such dosages.

Most of the quality research conducted to assess the health benefits of digestive enzymes has been performed in Europe using a product produced under the name Wobenzyme.

As a final note, there are herbal "bitters" (usually based upon extracts of *Gentiana lutea*) and other herbal digestive stimulants on the market. Some bitters are actually used as flavorings for drinks and in cooking.

Other Digestive Issues

Faulty carbohydrate metabolism is sometimes linked to intestinal invasion by the yeast *Candida albicans*. Those suspecting this problem should consult specialized literature, such as Scott J. Gregory *A Holistic Protocol for the Immune System* (1989), Luc De Schepper, *Candida* (1986) and *Peak Immunity* (1989). Approaches to controling yeast overgrowth include killing the yeast with products such as *nystatin,* citrus extract or other anti-yeast substances and supplementing the system with *L. acidophilus*, the much hardier bacteria *S. faecium 68* and other beneficial organisms. Beneficial bacterial products are avaialble through many different companies. As a rule, success in implanting friendly bacteria, such as *L.acidophilus*, in the face of a yeast overgrowth often requires the prior use of an anti-yeast product. A specialty bacterial strain,*Bacillus laterosporous* (B.O.D. strain), is recommended by Gregory, DeSchepper and some candida support groups for its anti-yeast benefits. Although considered effective for this purpose, *B. laterosporus* is presently the subject of considerable controversy.

#7
COENZYME Q_{10} (CoQ$_{10}$)

Anti-Fat Nutrient	CoQ$_{10}$
Fat Burning Function	Increases energy production at the cellular level.
Suggested Dose	30-60 mg in divided doses with meals.

COENZYME Q_{10} (CoQ$_{10}$)
In Depth

What Is It?

Coenzyme Q_{10} (CoQ$_{10}$), also called ubiquinone because it is present in nearly all cells, is obtained from the diet (mainly from fatty fish, organ meats, and whole grains) and is also produced by the body. Some have suggested that CoQ$_{10}$ will soon be classified as an oil-soluble vitamin because it is now known to be essential and because its deficiency leads to health problems. Chemically, its structure is related to that of the vitamins E and K. The amino acid methionine is essential for its production. CoQ$_{10}$ appears to be virtually non-toxic.

CoQ$_{10}$ is similar to L-carnitine in that it is important chiefly for its role in the mitochondria, the intracellular organelles which produce energy. The important energy storage chemical ATP (adenosine triphosphate) is produced by the mitochondria with the aid of CoQ$_{10}$. The coenzyme is also a potent antioxidant, as its structural similarity to vitamin E suggests. It quenches free radicals by donating its own electrons, and it also prevents lipid (fat) peroxidation in the body as do other antioxidants[36]

How CoQ$_{10}$ Helps With Weight Loss

As with L-carnitine, CoQ$_{10}$ may prove of benefit to those who are overweight because it improves the efficiency of energy production at the cellular level. There is some evidence that certain inefficiencies are related to genetic inheritances concerning the the body's ability to manufacture this coenzyme. About half of those with family histories of obesity do not respond to meals as they should. A normal response to a meal is for the body to slightly raise its rate of energy production. Many of those who are overweight do not have this response. Blood serum tests for levels of CoQ$_{10}$ indicate that these levels in almost 50% of the obese subjects were in fact deficient.[37]

OTHER BENEFITS OF CoQ$_{10}$

— Under the proper conditions it significantly improves athletic endurance.[38]

— It is used in Japan and elsewhere to treat congestive heart failure, cardiac arrhythmias and ischemic injury.[39]

— It is effective for lowering blood pressure.

— The coenzyme has been observed to serve as an immune stimulant which boosts the capacities of existing immune cells. It may reduce the toxic side effects of chemotherapy.

— Peridontal disease has been improved or even reversed with daily dosages of 50 to 70 mg.

How Is It Available and How Should It Be Taken?

CoQ_{10} is a relatively expensive supplement, or at least it has been until quite recently. It is available in 10, 30 and 60 mg. capsules. The effective amount is usually 10 to 20 mg. taken two or three times a day, although therapeutic dosages with heart patients have been as high as 150 mg. per day for four weeks or longer. Amounts of up to 100 mg. a day have been taken by Japanese purchasers for extended periods of time with only positive effects, so the safety of the coenzyme is well established. In Japan over 15 million people, about 10% of the entire population, take this coenzyme regularly. Some researchers suggest that additional benefits accrue if the CoQ_{10} is supplemented with 600 to 800 I.U. of vitamin E daily along with other basic nutrients.

#8

LIPOTROPICS

Anti-Fat Nutrients	Choline, Guggulipid and others.
Fat Burning Function	Dissolve and mobilize fat stores in the liver.
Suggested Dose	500-1500 mg in divided doses with meals.(choline)

LIPOTROPICS

In Depth

What Are They?

The primary site of lipotropic action is the liver. By definition, lipotropics serve to prevent the accumulation of fat in that organ, and they usually aid in the detoxification of metabolic wastes and other toxins. Some lipotropics help to emulsify fats so that these can be more readily transported by the blood. Other lipotropics work more directly with the digestion either by stimulating the liver to produce bile which is then sent to the gall bladder, or by stimulating the gall bladder to release its stored bile into the digestive tract to help emulsify fats.

Nutrient lipotropics include the amino acid methionine, the digestive aids betaine HCl and lipase (a fat digesting enzyme), and the substances choline and inositol. Herbal lipotropics include dandelion root, barberry, bearberry (*Arctostaphylos uva-ursa*), Oregon grape root, tumeric (*Curcumin*), milk thistle (*Silymarin*), wall germander (*Teucrium polium*) and many others. Several herbal lipotropics, including bearberry and tumeric, also act as insulin potentiators. Ancient Indian medical science, called

Ayurveda, lists the gum resin *guggul*, an extract from the guggul plant *(Commiphora mukul)* as a weight loss compound. It is typically used in conjunction with three special herbs to improve digestion and bowel function *(triphala)* or with *shilajit,* a mineral pitch noted for regulating blood sugar and liver disorders.

The special Ayurvedic compound guggul, standardized as Guggulipid (25 mg. guggulsterones per gram) has been shown to have a dramatic impact upon cholesterol and triglyceride levels, as well as being an aid to weight loss. Clinical studies have found that total cholesterol, LDL, VLDL and triglycerides all can be reduced by approximately 30% through the use of Guggulipid, yet the desirable HDL cholesterol fraction actually increases as much as 36% as a result of using this gum resin. When using the smaller amount of Guggulipid necessary for weight loss, these figures changed to 7-11% reductions for the bad blood fats and a 5-6% elevation of the good HDL. When using Ayurvedic weight loss formulas for a period of three months, non-dieting subjects lost 12.1 to 12.7 pounds more than did those taking a placebo.[40]

How Do Lipotropics Work?

In Chapter 5 it is noted that a significant number of those who are overweight also show signs of liver malfunctions. Lipotropics do not appear to have any significant impact upon lipolysis in athletes or in those of normal weight who are otherwise healthy.[41] However, they may be of use to those with special needs. In animal experiments, for instance, dandelion root extract served to dramatically reduce weight, although this was due partly to its action as a diuretic.[42] Choline may be a "conditionally essential" nutrient in that under conditions of high stress and/or in the absence of sufficient levels of methionine and perhaps folic acid, it is not manufactured in sufficient quantities by the body. In one study, healthy young adult men on a three week choline-free diet showed sharp declines of tissue concentrations of choline and a 50% increase of a blood serum marker of liver damage.

Some individuals report a reduction of fat and cellulite from the use of lipotropics. However, the biochemical explanations for such reports at this point are largely theoretical. Research suggests that supplementing with choline (20mg/kg body weight) may reduce body urinary carnitine losses as much as 75%. Also, it should be kept in mind that carnitne works synergistically with coenzyme Q_{10} and pantethine.[43]

Other Benefits of Lipotropics[44]

— Methionine and choline help detoxify the waste by-products of protein synthesis. This may be especially important for those on high protein diets.

— Lipotropics increase resistance to disease by stimulating the activity of the thymus gland.

— Choline, phosphatidyl choline, and other lipotropics can increase the production of lecithin in the liver.

— Lecithin may lower cholesterol levels and help to prevent cholesterol deposits. It may help to raise the desirable HDL blood levels.

— Lipotropics may be useful in preventing gallstone formation.

— Inositol has been shown to help protect the nerves in diabetic neuropathy.

— Silymarin and lipoic acid protect the liver against toxins, act as antioxidants and may improve the conversion of standard forms of vitamins, (e.g., B1 as thiamin HCl, B2 as riboflavin and so on, into their active co-enzyme forms: B1 as thiamine cocarboxylase, B2 as riboflavin 5' phosphate, etc.)

How Is It Available and How Should It Be Taken?

Each of the lipotropics mentioned above is available individually or in combination formulas. Effective doses for choline range from 500 to 1500mg in divided doses with meals. Recommended dosages for the other items are supplied by the manufacturers. The herbal lipotropics generally have even more pronounced effects than do choline and inositol. (Those taking methionine must always supplement with vitamin B-6 because this vitamin is required for the proper metabolism of this amino acid). *See also Special Responses in the Appendix page 138.*

Trials using Guggulipid alone without any other herbs indicated that as little as 200 mg. taken 3 times per day before meals caused weight loss in overweight subjects. The effective dosage may vary if combined with other ingredients, such as shilajit.

#9

DHEA

Anti-Fat Nutrient	DHEA
Fat Burning Function	Interferes with fat storage.
Suggested Dose	25-100 mg.

DHEA
(Dehydroepiandrosterone)
In Depth

What Is It?

DHEA is the primary steroid hormone produced by the adrenals and, in small amounts, by the testes. It possesses about 5% of the androgenic effect of testosterone. The body's production of DHEA increases until sometime in the 20s to a level of between 7 and 15 mg. of new production per day, and then declines gradually. By the age of 60, blood levels of the hormone typically are only two-thirds of those of early adulthood. By the age of 80, DHEA blood levels may have declined by 95%. Most of the DHEA within the body is found in the form of DHEA-S, that is, DHEA that has had a sulfate molecule attached to it by the liver. It is generally considered to be less active than is DHEA in most physiological processes. It may be possible to increase DHEA blood levels through dietary manipulation, but DHEA supplementation is best achieved with pharmaceutical-grade materials.

Technically, DHEA is a "pro-hormone" rather than an active hormone. It is the precursor to the steroid hormones of the body, including estrogen, progesterone, cortisone, testosterone and other steroid and sex hormones. DHEA can be converted to these otherwise difficult to construct hormones as needed, and any excess is simply excreted.[45]

How Does It Work?

Besides providing the building blocks for many of the body's most important hormones, DHEA works by inhibiting an enzyme called G6PD (glucose-6-phosphate dehydrogenase), which serves to store fat. The unstored fat is then either shunted into energy pathways or excreted. Obese individuals have been recognized as excreting less DHEA through the urine than do non-obese individuals, and this suggests that they are producing much less of this pro-hormone. Douglas L. Coleman and Edward H. Leiter of the Jackson Laboratory of Bar Harbor, Maine have found that very large doses of DHEA can apparently block or even reverse the effects of the genes responsible for obesity and diabetes in experimental animals. The blockage of G6PD may also explain the anti-tumor activity of DHEA in both animals and humans.[46]

DHEA is known to increase the insulin sensitivity of cells, an important factor in both diabetes and obesity. It also increases sensitivity to thyroid hormone, thus improving thermogenesis, fat metabolism and energy production. Finally, it improves liver function, thus ameliorating a weakness common to obese individuals.[47]

Unfortunately, animal models and experiments have yielded resulted which too often have not been reproduced in human trials. The clearest case is that of obesity, although there is quite a bit of controversy on this point. DHEA works extremely well in controlling obesity in rodents. Most human obesity trials, however, have proven successful only at very high levels of intake (1500 mg./day). Nevertheless, there is no doubt that DHEA is active against a range of conditions. Elderly patients given DHEA respond more favorably to flu vaccine. A study at the University of California, San Diego, reported recently in the national news found that aging subjects given this hormone precursor enjoyed "increased ability to cope with stress, increased quality of sleep, decreased joint pain, increased joint mobility and improved mood."

The human clinical evidence of DHEA's anti-obesity potential is spotty, although there is some data which suggests that the hormone has significant effects when used in conjunction with other weight-loss compounds. Two good published studies found no consistent results. In a study by Usiskin, *et al.*, no changes in body composition were demonstrated, even at 1600/mg. per day in obese men. Normal-weight men showed reduced body fat only for a brief time. A longer study by Morales, *et al.*, found no changes of significance in either men or women over a period of three months while using replacement levels of DHEA. Nevertheless, and albeit there are many individual exceptions, women who have the highest circulating levels of DHEA generally have the lowest body mass indexes.

Really good news for body builders and others who would like to increase lean tissue and reduce body fat with DHEA came out of a poster session at last year's New York Academy of Science's Conference on DHEA (June 18-19, 1995 at Washington, D.C.). D. Jakubowicz, *et al.*, of Venezuela, reported their results in a trial in which 300 mg. of DHEA was given nightly for one month to 22 men, ages 55-59. Insulin levels fell 27%, the growth-hormone-like IGF-1 increased 89%, body fat fell 14%, and lean tissue increased 7.8%. In the general discussion which closed the conference, Dr. Jorge Flechas maintained that although most people do not lose weight with DHEA, they do feel better and more vital, and men see a drop in LDL cholesterol and total cholesterol levels.

There are four ways in which DHEA may improve the lean-to-fat ratio of the body. These include influencing insulin levels and response, reducing food intake, reducing fat intake and increasing thermogenesis. A potential fifth mechanism is DHEA's effect upon cortisol levels in the body.[48] The first point is easy to document. DHEA levels are often inversely correlated with those of insulin, and this may be a reason why some individuals lose weight when they take the hormone. DHEA has been shown to increase the sensitivity of cells to insulin in humans.

Anecdotal reports exist to the effect that DHEA reduces food intake in humans. Unfortunately, the only real studies have been conducted with animals, specifically, with the Zucker obese rat. The inclusion of high doses of DHEA in the diets of these animals resulted in reductions in the amount of fat and protein which the animals voluntarily ate. After DHEA was removed from the diet, in at least one of the studies, the animals experienced rebound eating. Again, the implications for humans are not clear.

DHEA may increase thermogenesis by altering energy production in the liver. Most thermogenic compounds stimulate receptors, which are either beta-andrenergic agonists and/or alpha-antagonists. DHEA, however, appears to direct glucose utilization into an energy production pathway. This would account for at least some of the mood elevation and feelings of greater energy which are routinely reported with the use of DHEA. It also suggests once again that DHEA may be significant for weight loss only as part of a synergistic combination of compounds.

Finally, cortisol production provides an interesting marker for aging in that its secretion is inversely correlated with DHEA production. The ability to keep the synthesis of these hormones in balance and yet meet daily needs is called an *adaptive response* to the *stress response*. Most of the adaptive responses of the body decline markedly with age and with chronic stress, and aging and disturbances within the body's adaptive stress response clearly are closely linked. This connection has been explored by a number of researchers, amongst them Hans Selye. The stress response involves a feedback loop which links production of cortiotropic releasing hormone (CRH) provided by the hypothalamus to that of adrenocortiotropic hormone (ACTH) found in the pituitary gland to the release of corticosteroid hormones, such as cortisol, by the adrenal gland. Frequent and uncontrolled stress depletes DHEA levels — production is limited by the conversion rate from cholesterol — and disturbs the overall feedback mechanism between the adrenal cortex and the hypothalamus. Excessive cortisol production also causes a series of alterations in the general nature of the metabolism which, again, make a return to homeostasis more and more difficult. Elevated cortisol levels, of course, lead to the loss of lean tissues and, ultimately, to weight gain in many individuals.

Other Benefits of DHEA[49]

— Improves the symptoms of rheumatoid arthritis.

— May be a chemopreventative agent against cancer[50]

— May prevent or reverse some forms of diabetes.

— Enhances the functions of the immune system.

— Improves brain function.

— Protects against infections.

— May be a substitute for estrogen replacement.

— Exhibits life extension properties in laboratory animals.

How Is It Available and How Should It Be Taken?

It is sometimes claimed that DHEA is found in the Mexican wild yam, but most herbalists consider the Mexican yam to contain a pro-steroid compound which cannot be manipulated by human physiology to produce DHEA, although this pro-steroid can be synthetically altered to produce DHEA.

A dose of 50 mg. DHEA given at bedtime to men and women, aged 40-70, restored them to early adult blood levels within two weeks (Stanford University study). Some researchers maintain that DHEA is metabolized in the body within 8 hours. This suggests that taking divided doses of 25 mg. in the morning and the evening would be a preferred regimen, best taken before meals. There is no consensus available on dosage levels, other than that women should use only roughly half the dosage used by men because of size differences and because DHEA has very mild androgenic effects. In a lupus study utilizing 200 mg./day, half of the women reported acne, and some reported increased facial hair. In a similar study performed recently at Stanford University, a few women developed facial hair, even on dosages of 100 mg. However, many doctors report giving older women 50 mg./day routinely without side effects.

The majority of researchers consider DHEA supplementation to not be advisable for men and (especially) women below the age of 45 unless these are special reasons for its use. Dosages should be 10 to 50 mg. per day *for women*, depending upon age and other factors. *For men*, dosages should be between 25 and 100 mg. per day. *Dosages above these levels may cause androgenic effects in women and estrogenic effects in men.* Some doctors who specialize in sports medicine have reported that body builders using very high dosages of DHEA for extended periods of time have exhibited signs of elevated estrogen levels. Inasmuch as sex hormone production is closely regulated by the body, with each sex's primary pathway being the most closely regulated, it is possible to upregulate the alternate pathway.

The most promising area of potential benefit of DHEA for dieters is in a synergistic combination with other diet aids. Some studies have shown, for instance, that DHEA improves the efficacy of the diet drug fenfluramine when the two compounds are taken together. It is known that the brain, including the special region of the hypothalamus (which regulates appetite) has receptors for DHEA and/or DHEA metabolites. Fenfluramine alters levels of the brain chemical serotonin and specifically involves the hypothalamus, and this suggests that DHEA may influence satiety in conjunction with the same mechanisms. Therefore, DHEA may improve the effects of compounds which influence appetite and energy levels, even though DHEA, when used alone, has only a mild effect upon body weight. For other benefits found with DHEA, the reader is advised to consult *DHEA: A Practical Guide* by Ray Sahelian (Avery, 1996).

WARNING

Men with enlarged prostates or prostatic cancer and women with reproductive cancers, breast cancer of endometriosis should avoid DHEA. The conditions, which are stimulated by androgens and estrogens, may be stimulated by the androgenic aspects of DHEA. However, there is no consensus to date regarding the effects of DHEA upon sex hormone sensitive cancers.

#10
FIBER

Anti-Fat Nutrient	Fiber
Fat Burning Function	Reduces appetite, reduces fat absorption and more.
Suggested Dose	2-4 capsules before meals with extra water.

FIBER
In Depth

What Is It?

Fiber exists in soluble, semisoluble and insoluble forms. Insoluble fibers are those for which humans lack digestive enzymes, and therefore they do not break down significantly in our digestive tracts. Cellulose from grain brans, some parts of fruits and vegetables, and lignin from legumes are insoluble fibers. These fibers provide roughage to insure bowel movements.

Soluble fibers, which do break down under the action of our digestive enzymes, include pectins and gums (mucilages). About a third of the fiber in fruits, vegetables, and many legumes is soluble. Some grains, such as oats and barley, contain large amounts of soluble fibers. These are considered highly desirable fibers. Pectins have long been known to promote wound healing, to slow the absorption of glucose from the intestines into the blood stream, to bind a number of toxic chemicals thus preventing their absorption, and to aid in the reduction of cholesterol levels through the binding of bile acids.[51]

Hemicellulose has qualities of both insoluble and soluble fibers. Psyllium husks, the dried seed coat of the Indian native *Plantago ovata*, is perhaps the best of these. It acts as roughage and absorbs and removes toxins from the intestines. It also moistens and soothes irritated intestinal membranes.

How Fiber Helps With Weight Loss

It is now recognized that the addition of fiber to the diet, especially soluble and semi-soluble fibers, offers many health benefits. Mixtures of sources of fibers of various types can be designed to work together synergistically to maximize their health-promoting properties. They act to regularize bowel functions, including the control of both diarrhea and constipation, to soothe irritated mucous membranes in the gastrointestinal tract, and to absorb various toxins and bacteria, which are then eliminated with the help of the bulking action of the fibers. Psyllium husks have long been used in traditional medical systems, such as that of the Indian/Ayurvedic tradition, to perform precisely these functions.[52] As already noted, they have properties of both soluble and non-soluble fibers, but do not produce the gas and bloating nor the intestinal irritation characteristic of crude fibres, such as wheat bran.[53]

Fiber plays an important role in helping to reduce excess weight. The bulk of the fiber itself gives a physical sensation of fullness which helps to control how much is eaten at a given meal. Appetite is reduced directly by the bulk of the fiber and indirectly through the delayed emptying of the stomach and the release of brain and gastrointestinal tract hormones which signal satiety.[54]

The bulking action of soluble fibers significantly slows the release of carbohydrates into the blood from the intestines. The limited post-meal rise in blood sugar levels associated with the consumption of complex carbohydrates, especially with those of vegetables and legumes, likewise moderates the release of insulin into the blood and avoids both the health dangers and the surges in appetite which characterize the body's responses to excessive insulin release.[55] Some have suggested that adding fiber to meals can help reduce the impact of carbohydrates on the glycemic response.[56]

Just how important is dietary fiber in controlling weight? One recent study found that lean individuals eat about 50% more fiber than do those who are either moderately or severely obese. The amount of fiber in the diets of the three groups was estimated to be 18.8 grams versus 13.3 grams versus 13.7 grams, respectively. Other significant roles for fiber include the lowering of total cholesterol and the reduction of the incidence of colorectal cancer. People who consume the most fiber have 47% less colorectal cancer and 66% less pancreatic cancer than those who eat the least fiber.[57] Since colon cancer ranks just behind lung cancer as a cause of death, the protection afforded by fiber against this particular cancer is of considerable importance.[58]

How Is It Available and How Should It Be Taken?

The preferred sources of fiber are the soluble and semi-soluble varieties. Pectin, guar gum, oat bran, barley and psyllium seed husks are such sources. Some of the new fiber products made from citrus sources may also come under this heading of preferred fibers. Whole foods can supply significant amounts of fiber. Oats, barley, oat bran, and various legumes can be added to the diet on a regular basis to supply sufficient quantities of these fiber groups. However, if this is not possible, the more concentrated of these fibers are available in tablets, capsules and powdered/granulated forms. Two to four tablets/capsules or one or two teaspoons of granules/powder can be taken an hour before meals. These dosages should always be taken with at least eight or more ounces of water or serious dehydration can result.

CAUTION

Although most of us can probably benefit from adding fiber to our diets, too much of a good thing, including fiber, can create problems. This is especially true of the insoluble fibers such as wheat bran. Fiber also can be hard on the intestines if taken in excess. Some symptoms of excess fiber consumption are bloating, diarrhea and nausea. Moreover, just as fiber can absorb toxins from the colon, most types of fiber can interfere with the absorption of some nutrients. Therefore, it may be a good idea to take fiber supplements at a different time than when you take your meals or your vitamin and mineral supplements.

#11
THERMOGENIC AIDS

Anti-Fat Nutrient	Ephedra and others.
Fat Burning Function	Increase metabolic rate, suppress the appetite.
Suggested Dose	100 mg with breakfast and lunch.

THERMOGENIC AIDS
In Depth

What Are They?

Thermogenesis is an increase in the body's production of heat-energy triggered by nutritional and biochemical means. One of the chief drawbacks of calorie-restricted diets is their tendency to lower the body's rate of energy production. Thermogenic aids can help correct this. Common aids include caffeine, L-phenylalanine, L-tyrosine, the Chinese herb ma huang, L-carnitine and other products.

How Thermogenics Help With Weight Loss

As we will discuss in Chapter 5, individuals prone to obesity often have lower basal metabolic rates (BMR), and obesity itself promotes a lowering of the BMR. After eating, most people see a lasting rise in energy production amounting to 10-20% of their prior metabolic rates. For reasons not well understood, overweight women in particular do not experience this increase in heat production.[59]

Certain naturally occurring substances, such as ephedrine contained in the herb ma huang, speed up the resting metabolic rate, act as mild stimulants and tend to suppress the appetite. Caffeine and other members of the xanthine family have similar effects, and can be found in coffee, kola nut, tea, yerbamate, and many other herb teas and foods. The seaweed known as bladderwrack (fucus) also activates the thyroid and has been used in Europe to treat obesity and hypothyroidism since the 17th century.

Many of the substances listed in the section above on appetite suppressants also act to raise the metabolic rate. L-phenylalanine and L-tyrosine perform this function by serving as precursors to epinephrine and norepinephrine, that is, as precursors to adrenaline and noradrenaline. High-protein diets, which supply these amino acids, will tend to speed up bodily processes in general. Since thyroid activators often produce results similar to adrenal stimulants, the following section on the thyroid is also important. Thyroid hormone and norepinephrine both activate brown fat. Also of great importance (see Chapter Five) is the need to prevent the suppression of the action of the lipolytic and brown fat activating hormone *glucagon* by insulin (released by the consumption of carbohydrates).

(Caffeine, ephedrine and related products should not be consumed in excess. They make susceptible individuals nervous and activate a feedback circuit involving the thyroid.)

New studies have revealed yet another thermogenic herb, or rather a new use for an old substance. It seems that Yohimbine hydrochloride, an extract from the bark of the yohimbe tree, not only is at least partially the male sexual stimulant which tradition claims that it is, but is also able to increase the release of noradrenalin. This action "stimulates the system, raises body temperature, and causes the body to mobilize fat for fuel. Yohimbine appears to be effective in all these areas."[60] In one study patients given 15 mg. of yohimbe hydrochloride a day on a 1000 calorie a day diet lost an average of 7.8 pounds in three weeks in comparison with 4.8 pounds lost by the controls.[61] There are other thermogenic aids in the plant kingdom as well, such as mustard seed and cayenne pepper. These last two items help to begin the thermogenic process and make other substances, including caffeine and ephedrine, more effective as thermogenic aids.

Caffeine and ephedrine work better together than does either alone. Ephedrine mimics many of the effects of the release of adrenaline from the adrenal glands. Caffeine, which stimulates the pituitary directly and the thyroid indirectly, stimulates the adrenals through the action of the thyroid. The theophylline found in tea also opens up the peripheral capillaries to a certain extent. This means that the heat generated by thermogenesis can be dissipated. Fat acts as an insulator and thereby usually causes the body to turn off heat production. Some diet formulas add additional anti-pyretics such as aspirin or white willow bark in order to further dissipate the heat produced by thermogenic stimulants. Anti-pyretics are essential for safe thermogenesis. Antioxidants, likewise, are necessary for the safe long-term use of thermogenic products inasmuch as such stimulation increases free radical production. Interestingly, the antioxidant polyphenols found in tea, such as the catechins, and not just the caffeine and theophylline, also may improve thermogenesis. It has been known for 30 years that catechins slow the destruction of the body's adrenaline. Now it has been shown in tissue studies that tea extracts alone stimulate thermogenesis in brown fat and that the effect is stronger when ephedrine is added.[62]

However, the action of the adrenal stimulants can be increased indirectly through supplements that contain the building blocks for adrenal hormones, for example L-tyrosine. This approach has the advantage of helping to prevent thyroid and adrenal exhaustion. Exhaustion of the sympathetic nervous system can be avoided through the addition of hawthorne berry, licorice and magnesium to formulas. The health of the adrenal glands and the parasympathetic nervous system can be safeguarded by the addition of acetylcholine precursors such as DMAE(dimethylaminoethanol) and vitamin B5(pantothenic acid or its coenzyme pantethine).

Availablity and Usage

Thermogenic aids have become quite common as diet aids. They work so successfully that pharmaceutical research is now being directed toward this approach to weight loss. A new class of drugs called thermogenic beta-3 agonists is being developed in Europe to perform as thermogenic aids. However, these are not expected to be available until the end of this decade.[63]

Yohimbe products are available, but most are lacking in the active ingredient. As with all herbs, only buy products with guaranteed potencies or other forms of standardization.

CAUTIONS

No strong stimulants should be used by those with high blood pressure, thyroid imbalances, heart irregularities or similar problems. Women with fibrocystic breast disease should avoid xanthines as these may aggravate this condition. Caution should be exercised in mixing sources of caffeine and ephedrine, or these two with L-phenylalanine or L-tyrosine. Taken together in excess, these combinations can lead to nervousness, excitability, insomnia and nausea. Morever, long term usage of large amounts of adrenal mimics and stimulants may be undesirable, especially in the absence of nutrients which support this gland's health and that of the nervous system. (See Anti-Fat Nutrient #17 for the thyroid.) Traditional systems of herbal treatment commonly add herbs such as licorice and hawthorne to strong stimulant formulas in order to reduce negative side effects. Thermogenesis inducers should be cycled 5-6 days on and 1-2 days off per week and also 3 weeks on and 1 week off per month. *See also Special Responses in the Appendix page 138.*

WARNING

In September 1992 the FDA issued an import bulletin on the herb ephedra. The attempt is being made to reclassify ephedra from a food to an "unapproved food additive." Although no ban is yet in place, that may be the next step. Legal questions arise regarding the FDA's action in this case because related compounds and extracts are freely sold over-the-counter in many cold and sinus medications, and many varieties of the herb have long been used in teas.

#12

MCT's

Anti-Fat Nutrient	MCT's
Fat Burning Function	Increase burning of calories.
Suggested Dose	2-4 grams total before or after workouts with meals.

MCT's (Medium-Chain Triglycerides)
In Depth

What Are They?

MCT's have been used for many years for special purposes. MCT's are sometimes found in the nutrient mixtures of bedridden patients dependent upon intravenous nutrition. They were developed in part because they do not require the action of bile for digestion, but are absorbed directly through the walls of the small intestine and transported to the liver for oxidation. (As structurally alterred fats, they have several carbon atoms removed from the normal structure of the long-chain triglycerides).

How MCT's Burn Fat

In seriously catabolic patients, MCT's were found to help prevent the body from depleting its lean and muscle tissues. Moreover, MCT's are not stored as bodyfat, but rather they are preferentially burned in the mitochondria of the cells to provide energy.[64] For some athletes and bodybuilders, this quality has proved useful since excess training depletes the glycogen stores of the muscles, and continued training after that point can only take place partially through the break down of muscle protein for fuel. Extreme endurance athletes do not just burn fat; they burn muscle as well.

Does this mean that MCT's can help dieters? Yes, as long as there are not too many expectations. MCT's do seem to promote lipolysis (fat burning) and they appear to have a pronounced thermogenic effect.[65] Nevertheless, actual studies with clinically obese subjects have proved disappointing. The subjects lost weight, but at about the same rate as on other similar low calorie diets. The thermogenic and lipolytic aspects of MCT's seem to be more significant for healthy subjects of normal weight and for those moderately overweight than for those who are clinically obese. However, MCT's do serve to protect the body's protein in the lean tissues during the use of low calorie and low carbohydrate diets.[66]

How Are They Available and How Should They Be Taken?

MCT's contain about 118 calories per tablespoonful and can be added to a variety of foods in place of oils and fats. Since MCT's can cause stomach upset and diarrhea if taken in too large quantities, the dieter should begin with no more than a tablespoonful. Also, these *are* still fats, even if structurally altered ones. In those with liver problems, quantities of MCT's taken on an empty stomach may raise blood lipids. Finally, like any other fat or oil, MCT's are subject to oxidation and should be taken with with antioxidants.

The FDA recognizes MCT's only as nutrients. They are available in many health food stores, primarily in the sports supplements sections. A few companies offer MCT Oil and suggest its use in cooking, as a salad dressing or by the spoonfull from the bottle in small amounts It is available in bottles of 90 capsules of 1 gram each and as a 16 fluid ounce liquid.

#13
LIPOGENESIS INHIBITORS

Anti-Fat Nutrient	(—)–Hydroxycitric Acid (HCA)
Fat Burning Function	Decreases fat production and storage.
Suggested Dose	1500 mg to several grams in divided doses with meals.

LIPOGENESIS INHIBITORS ˉ
(Inhibitors of Fat Production and Storage)
In Depth

What Are They?

Inhibitors of lipogenesis are substances which slow the production of fats from the metabolism of carbohydrates and proteins. This means inhibiting, for instance, the synthesis of triglycerides and/or cholesterol. Some known drugs, such as Triton, inhibit lipogenesis, but these drugs typically have side effects and they rapidly lose effectiveness with continued use. Fortunately, safe and effective natural alternatives are now being discovered. One such natural alternative is (—)–hydroxycitric acid, which also is called (—)–hydroxycitrate or HCA. HCA is extracted primarily from the dried pericarp (rind) of the fruit of *Garcinia cambogia*, a native plant of South Asia popularly used in cooking, including the preparation of curries. Aside from food preparation, *G. cambogia* is used as a preservative, as a purgative for the treatment of intestinal worms and parasites, and for bilious digestive conditions.[67] Traditionally, *G. cambogia* is said to aid the digestion and to make meals more "filling."

How HCA Blocks Fat

HCA is remarkable for its ability to reduce the body's own synthesis of fats. During the normal metabolism of meals, carbohydrate calories which are neither used immediately for energy nor stored as glycogen are converted into fats in the liver by the enzyme ATP-citrate lyase. HCA inhibits this enzyme, and by doing so it also reduces the formation of acetyl coenzyme A, a biochemical which plays a key role in carbohydrate and fat metabolism. As a result, the production of low density lipoprotein (LDL) and triglycerides is inhibited. The net effect is that fat production and storage is reduced. The appetite is controlled, food consumption is cut and thermogenesis may be enhanced.[68]

HCA is a substance which has been studied extensively for a period of more than two decades. Numerous animal trials conducted at major universities and described in peer-reviewed journals have demonstrated both the safety and the efficacy of HCA in inhibiting the production of fats from carbohydrate calories. The results of these trials have been so impressive that one of the world's largest pharmaceutical firms, Hoffmann-La Roche, not only sponsored much of the work, but also has sought synthetic versions of HCA which it can patent and market as diet aids. To date, no such synthetic products are available.

Because HCA has been so extensively studied, it is possible to distinguish among the various extracts available on the market. Quality control is of major importance since the desired effect is dosage-dependent. As it turns out, it is quite difficult to establish the exact amount of HCA present in an extract. Many companies which claim to have a concentration of 50% HCA actually have mistakenly counted tartaric, citric and other organic acids present in the rind as part of the HCA content. Also important is the form of HCA used. In animal trials, the lactone form of HCA has proven less effective than the salt form. According to data from Hoffman-La Roche, the rate of conversion of free HCA in solution into its lactone is approximately 10% per week at low room temperature.

How Is It Available and How Should It Be Taken?

Since all *Garcinia* products on the market are extracts and not pure HCA, consumers should look for the actual HCA content. For instance, 500 mg. of a true and verified HCA will provide 250 mg. of HCA. The effective dosage of actual HCA probably begins at 500 mg. taken 2 to 3 times per day in conjunction with a low fat/low alcohol, high complex carbohydrate diet. For most individuals 1500 mg of HCA is a good starting dosage. If desired results are not seen within three weeks the dosage should be doubled and may be increased up to a total of 5-6 grams per day. Adequate water must be consumed while taking HCA. Some individuals may experience loose stool during the first week at higher dosages of HCA, but this will pass as the intestinal flora adjusts. HCA is several times more effective when taken two or three times per day one half-hour to one hour before meals than when taken only once per day. The product likewise may work better when combined with chromium and/or other insulin potentiators and mimics.

In Asia, the fruit of *Garcinia* species is used to make a soup which is eaten before meals for weight loss. Although the usual recommendation is that HCA in tablets and capsules should be taken 30 to 60 minutes *before* meals with a glass of water or with mid-morning and mid-afternoon fruit snacks, Asian usage suggests that taking HCA three times a day *with* meals may make a good approach. Dieters who do not find good results with the usual method should try taking HCA with each meal. Moreover, a bowl of light soup before lunch and supper does seem to make HCA work better. HCA increases the body's own satiety signal, so it is best to slow down how quickly meals are eaten. This strategy gives the body a chance to signal that enough has been eaten. Never skip meals and do not take HCA in place of a meal — it requires food to work. Those who are sensitive to citric acid (i.e., to oranges, tomatoes, etc.) may be sensitive to *Garcinia* extracts as well.

Again, most people need at least 1500 mg. of HCA (3 grams of a 50% material) divided into two or three equal doses to get consistent results. The best recent evidence suggests that the newly available HCA *potassium* salts are both much more effective and more effective for a greater percentage of users than are the HCA calcium salts. (See the review in the June 1996 issue of *Let's Live*.) Liquid *Garcinia* extracts likewise appear to be more readily absorbed, although not to the extent seen with the potassium salts. Concurrent use of the nutrient L-carnitine may improve results, especially when the fat content of the diet is not closely regulated.

HCA in the form of the calcium salt when used alone will not prevent binge eating and appears to work best in conjunction with other dietary measures. Most of the studies performed with HCA were designed to avoid binge eating patterns, and included more water and vegetables and less fat than are typical of the usual American diet. Under these conditions and when enough of the compound was ingested according to directions, HCA consistently has produced moderate weight loss. When used in conjunction with a calorie-restricted diet (1200 kcal/day), roughly 1500 mg. of HCA per day typically leads to about 60% greater weight loss than is found with a placebo, i.e., 14 pounds versus 8 pounds over an 8 week period. Results without such measures have been less consistent. However, new HCA products (probably under patent) will soon appear on the market, which work well without the necessity of detailed attention to diet. In a recent pilot test undertaken in East Asia, one such product led to an average weight loss of 1.5 pounds per week *without* any changes in the daily diet on the part of test subjects. In other words, the new HCA compound led to as much weight loss without calorie restriction as does calcium HCA as part of a restricted calorie diet.

#14
ANTIOXIDANTS

Anti-Fat Nutrient	Vitamin C, Beta-Carotene and others.
Fat Burning Function	Help detoxify the waste products of fat metabolism.
Suggested Dose	Dosages vary, see below.

ANTIOXIDANTS
In Depth

What Are They?

Antioxidants are substances which remove the by-products of oxidative and similar reactions from the body. A simple example of an oxidative reaction is our everyday metabolism. When our body burns food for energy, it takes oxygen molecules from the air and reacts these with molecules of carbohydrates, proteins and fats. If the chemical reaction is complete or "clean," then only water, carbon dioxide and heat are produced. However, the burning process often is not complete, and even when it is, the oxygen which it requires will readily react chemically with parts of the body other than food sources of energy. The result is the creation of what are known as "free radicals." These molecules are highly reactive because they have at least one unpaired electron which they seek to balance by reacting with another molecule. On the one hand, nutrients which are antioxidants very easily donate electrons to or combine with free radicals, thus preventing the radicals from doing damage to the body's tissues. On the other hand, the antioxidants themselves do not become chemically reactive after having "quenched" free radicals, and they either are easily removed from the body or are easily restored back to their original condition.

Free radicals damage the tissues in several ways. Perhaps the most direct is their attack on the membranes of cells. Cell membranes consist of proteins and lipids (fats). Free radicals can break the strands of proteins, cause the lipids to link to one another, and improperly bind the proteins and the lipids in other ways.. This damage prevents the cell from properly taking in nutrients and from properly removing waste products. The symptom commonly used to illustrate the results of free radical attack on the membranes of cells is the loss of elasticity characteristic of aged skin. Yet damage to the wall of the cell is nevertheless preferable to mischief done within the cell itself, for free radical activity inside the cell can alter the replication of the DNA and thereby initiate cancerous changes.[69]

Antioxidants come in three primary forms. The most important are enzymes which are produced by the cells themselves. These include superoxide dismutase (SOD), catalase and glutathione peroxidase. Of secondary importance, but easier to use as supplements, are the non-enzymatic antioxidants which are vitamins. These include vitamin A and its safer form as beta-carotene, vitamin C, vitamin E and a large number of less easily classifiable items, such as various flavonoids and polyphenols derived from citrus fruits, red wine, green tea, and so on. Also in this category are the substances L-Carnitine and Coenzyme Q_{10} (CoQ_{10}). A third category of antioxidants consists of certain minerals which are required in minute quantities and which include zinc and selenium. These minerals work mostly as co-factors of the vitamins and as actual components of the primary antioxidant enzymes.

For years, evidence has been accumulating which indicates that many antioxidants may improve the body's response to insulin. This has been demonstrated for the vitamins C and E, and for many of the flavonoids and polyphenols derived from fruits and vegetables. Tea Catechins and similar compounds may also increase the rate of thermogenesis. (See the section on Thermogenic

Aids.) Individuals who want to improve their blood sugar levels and to improve their response to their body's own insulin might try taking 1 to 3 grams of vitamin C and 400 to 800 I.U. of vitamin E per day.

How Antioxidants Help With Weight Loss

As a dieter loses weight, the body is forced to burn fats. To stay healthy while your body is burning fat at an accelerated rate, you should add antioxidants to your diet. Fat burning creates metabolic waste products which include ketones and lipid peroxides. Peroxides are themselves free radicals. Perhaps even more damaging are the oil-soluble toxins and pesticides from the industrial environment which collect in the body's fat stores. These include residues of DDT, PCB's, lindane, chlordane and other noxious chemicals. All of these stored toxins are released as the dieter loses weight by burning fats, although they are much more easily removed from the body if exercise is a part of the process. Many of them are directly implicated as damaging to the body's ability to metabolize fats for energy, as themselves promoting the formation of free radicals, and so forth.[70] None of these waste products of fat metabolism or toxins and pesticides released through the diet will make the dieter feel better. On the contrary, they will interfere with weight loss and they will certainly contribute to fatigue and other discomforts associated with dieting. By now there is a massive amount of research which indicates that supplements such as vitamin C and E are useful in controlling free radicals and in preventing or treating ailments such as arthritis, cancer, diabetes and heart disease.[71] The dieter should also be aware that the use of anorectics and thermogenic aids, both of which tend to speed up the body, will increase the production of free radicals and therefore the need for antioxidants.

How Are They Available and How Should They Be Taken?

There are many nutrient formulas which include antioxidants among their vitamins and minerals. Those individuals undertaking rigorous and stressful programs such as dieting commonly find the addition to the diet of larger than RDA amounts to be helpful. Vitamin C usually is suggested at dosages of 2 grams or more a day in a non-acidic form divided among all the meals taken. Vitamin E is useful in dosages of 400-800 IU, although as an oil-soluble vitamin it probably should not be taken in excess of 800 IU per day. (Only the natural d-alpha tocopheryl and other more minor natural forms of vitamin E appear to be active in the body as antioxidants.)[72] Similarly, vitamin A, which is oil-soluble and toxic at high dosages, is usually most safely taken in the form of beta-carotene, which is non-toxic even at high dosages. Typical doses for beta-carotene range from 25,000 to 50,000 units.

Dosages of the newer (and often far more powerful) antioxidants vary according to the manufacturers' instructions and according to your needs as well as your budget. The extract of pine bark known as pycnogenol and the closely related grape seed extracts are hundreds of times as powerful as vitamin C, but also many times more expensive. Furthermore, the absorption and the effectiveness of some of the best antioxidants is greatly improved if these antioxidants are taken in conjunction with other items. For instance, the highly potent bioflavonoid Quercitin is much better absorbed by the body if taken on an empty stomach with the proteolytic enzyme bromelain (see the section of digestive enzymes earlier.)

Antioxidants work best when used in conjunction with a well balanced vitamin and mineral formula and with the proper diet. Note: The dieter who chooses to use large dosages of supplements of any sort and who later wants to cut back is advised to reduce the supplement(s) over a period of time to avoid any rebound effect.

#15
GRAPEFRUIT PILLS

Anti-Fat Nutrient	Grapefruit, teas, and others.
Fat Burning Function	Increase fat excretion from the body, are diuretics, etc.
Suggested Dose	Dosages vary.

GRAPEFRUIT AND OTHER
FAT-LOSS PRODUCTS
In Depth

Grapefruit

Grapefruit has been used as a weight loss aid for many years. This citrus fruit is high in pectin, a soluble fiber which lowers cholesterol and increases the amount of fat excreted from the body. Some studies involving pectin have shown that it markedly increases the amount of fat removed from the body. (See the foregoing section on fiber.) As a whole fruit, grapefruit provides vitamins, some minerals, much roughage, but very few calories. It also helps to correct the acid balance of the blood. As an aid to weight loss, it may deserve some of the reputation that it has. However, it does not work miracles. Grapefruit in pill form offers few benefits.

Starch Blocker

Starch Blocker received a great deal of attention a few years ago. It is yet another product which the FDA ordered removed from the marketplace. Starch Blocker contains the protein *phaseolamin*, which interferes with the digestion of starch. Consequently, it prevents the calories from starch from being absorbed. There is always a downside to any action which prevents normal digestion, so it may be fortunate starch blocker is off the market. For those seeking sustainable weight loss and improved health, a better course of action is to add nutrients and fiber to the diet, and to correct the imbalances which originally resulted in the gain of unwanted pounds.

Meal Replacement Formulas

See the general discussion in Chapter 5. There are now many diets and diet systems which involve replacing one or two meals a day with a liquid or a powdered drink mix. These 90-300 calorie formulas usually contain one third of the RDA of vitamins, minerals and various ratios of protein and carbohydrates. Keep in mind that it is not recommended to drop below 800 calories per day on any diet program, *and the lower the number of calories, the greater the need for high quality protein.* Well designed formulas provide the proper amount of quality protein necessary for a very low calorie diet. The best-selling brands at the supermarket rarely provide either enough protein or protein of high enough quality because high quality protein is costly. Indeed, the major ingredients of the most heavily promoted national brands often are sugars.

Meal replacement programs are generally expensive, lack adequate fiber and suffer from the various drawbacks discussed in Chapter 5.

Weight Loss Teas

Teas which act upon the liver are discussed under Lipotropics. Teas which increase thermogenesis are discussed under Thermogenic Aids. Other weight loss teas contain herbs which produce laxative or diuretic effects upon the body. Some of the more complex formulas include herbs which curb the appetite and interfere with fat digestion. Simple diuretics should be avoided as a way to lose weight.

Apple Cider Vinegar, Kelp, B-6, Lecithin Combinations

These formulas were among the first to address weight loss at the biochemical level. Kelp contains iodine, which nourishes the thyroid gland and can raise the basal metabolic rate if the thyroid is underactive due to a lack of this mineral. Vitamin B-6 is necessary for fat metabolism, has diuretic properties, and its deficiency plays a role in some types of diabetes. Lecithin contains some lipotropic nutrients, *but only if the lecithin is of the very highest quality.* Most soy lecithin is of little use for nutritional purposes. Apple cider vinegar is reputed to have thyroid-stimulating and fat-emulsifying properties. These formulas likely have a small impact under circumstances of deficiencies of basic nutrients, but greater and more consistent results require more complete nutrient formulas.

#16
DHA AND PYR
(Dihydroxyacetone and Pyruvate)

Anti-Fat Nutrient	DHA and PYR
Fat Burning Function	Provides extra energy on low carbohydrate diets.
Suggested Dose	See manufacuturers recommendations.

DHA AND PYR
(Dihydroxyacetone and Pyruvate)
In Depth

What Are They?

These two compounds are linked to carbohydrate metabolism in the body. Through oxidation they increase the body's energy reserves of ATP. ATP (adenosine triphosphate) exists within cells, especially muscle cells. DHA is at the present better known for its use in cosmetics[73] than in dieting, although that may change. The oxidation of both compounds is quite complex within the body's basic energy cycle called the Krebs cycle. The taste of the powders is slightly sweet.

How Do They Work?

DHA and PYR are mentioned here because they have proven useful in some studies of very-low-calorie diets (VLCD's). These are diets consisting of between 400 and 800 calories, and usually using 40-50 grams of high quality protein. Going below 800 calories probably adds no additional weight loss benefit. VLCD's work best if some small number of calories from carbohydrates are consumed, for otherwise the dieter's own protein tissue will be broken down to support blood glucose levels for the brain.

In one study, women followed a liquid diet of 500 calories a day with 60% of the calories from carbohydrates and less than 1 gram of fat. The subjects were given either DHA or PYR, whereas controls received a glucose polymer. After three weeks, both weight and total fat losses were greater with those taking DHA or PYR. Protein-sparing was the same as in the controls. Also, there is some indication that the use of DHA and PYR in VLCDs (and afterwards) may reduce the rebound gain of weight and fat stores when the diet is ended.[74] No major side effects have been discovered in the limited studies thus far conducted.

Many years ago, it was discovered the pyruvate added to the diet prevented alcohol from causing animals to develop fatty livers. This suggested that the compound might have a generally positive effect on the functioning of the liver. Pyruvate is now covered by a large number of U.S. patents describing its use for weight loss, lowering blood fats, reducing insulin levels, increasing glycogen stores and, most recently, preventing free radical generation. In animal studies, pyruvate has been shown to increase both thermogenesis and general energy expenditure. Even the rate of synthesis of new fat in fat cells appears to be affected by pyruvate, although the reasons for this are unclear.

The major drawback with the use of pyruvate in weight loss is, as already noted, the large amount required. The dosage listed in the patents runs from 2 to 15% of the total calories in the diet, and this presumes the concurrent ingestion of a low fat diet. Translated into human dietary terms, this means the lower threshold of intake for proven efficacy with pyruvate is about 10 grams per day under good conditions and ranges up to 50 grams. Whether this threshold can be lowered and the proven benefits of pyruvate increased through other means is still being explored. A soon-to-be-published article in the *International Journal of Obesity* suggests that dosages in the range of 6 grams may prove effective. (See U.S. Patents 4,812,479; 4,874,790; 5,134,162 and 5,480,909.) However, this 6 gram dosage is based upon extrapolations from changes in animal response curves and not upon human data.

Availability and Usage

Pyruvate has recently become available for use in diet products. The version in which pyruvate is stabilized with calcium is preferable to the one stabilized with sodium, so purchasers should read the fine print and look for the ingredient "calcium pyruvate." Instructions for use will be found on the products.

#17
THYROID ACTIVATORS

Anti-Fat Nutrients	L-Tyrosine, Iodine and others.
Fat Burning Function	Nourish the thyroid gland.
Suggested Dose	Ideally taken in combination with other nutrients, see below.

THYROID NUTRIENTS
AND ACTIVATORS
In Depth

The Importance Of The Thyroid

The thyroid is an endocrine gland located in the neck. It produces two hormones, *thyroxine* and *triiodothyronine*, which are responsible for various functions in the body. These hormones increase protein synthesis in all body tissues and they increase the activity of NA/K ATPase enzymes. These latter enzymes influence the rate at which fat is burned for energy. If the thyroid is not functioning properly, a slow metabolism can result. Thus, many people with underactive thyroids also have weight problems. Thyroid dysfunction also is often involved in menstrual difficulties.

A common method for testing thyroid function is to place a thermometer under the arm for ten minutes before getting out of bed in the morning. The thermometer must read to tenths of a degree. Normal body temperature ranges for this test are between 97.8 and 98.2 degrees Fahrenheit.

Readings below 97.8 may indicate hypothyroid activity (low thyroid), and readings above may indicate hyperthyroid activity (excess thyroid).

Some of the factors which can cause thyroid problems (thereby decreasing the rate at which the body burns calories) include malnourishment of the thyroid through vitamin and mineral deficiencies, thyroid and/or pituitary exhaustion as a result of overstimulation with caffeine, sugar and other stimulants, and the presence of substances which inhibit thyroid function, such as alcohol.

Care Of The Thyroid Gland and Its Role In Obesity

Most people associate the thyroid gland with iodine, and iodine is important. However, thyroid functioning benefits from good nutrition in general. Deficiencies of vitamin A, B-2, C and E have all been linked to thyroid insufficiency. Moreover, there is a link between thyroid malfunction and the inability either to absorb some nutrients or to transform others into their active forms. Vitamin B-12 is an example of the first and the transformation of beta-carotene into vitamin A is an example of the second.[75] Since the use of supplemental thyroid hormones requires the supervision of a doctor, this is a case in which an ounce of prevention is worth a pound of cure.

The thyroid's regulatory function is commonly damaged through the excessive consumption of caffeine, sugar and other simple carbohydrates. These act as pituitary stimulants, and the pituitary, in turn, stimulates the release of thyroid hormones. Excessive stimulation of the pituitary ultimately damages that gland's ability to produce the hormone necessary to activate the thyroid, whereas serotonin, the hormone which reduces thyroid activity, continues to be produced.

Whatever the source of hypothyroidism, the effects are the same. Inadequate thyroid hormone secretion causes the adrenal glands to fail to secrete enough cortisol. Without adrenal cortisol, the liver does not produce and store enough glycogen, an essential storage sugar which the liver releases in a controlled manner to maintain balanced blood sugar levels. As a result, hypothyroidism can lead to a feeling of sluggishness and lassitude as well as to craving for sugars and other simple carbohydrates.[76]

A good thyroid support formula should combine L-tyrosine (a precursor to the thyroid hormones) with the following: magnesium, potassium, zinc, manganese, iodine, vitamin B-1 (thiamine), vitamin B-2 (riboflavin), vitamin B-3 (niacin), vitamin B-6, and the antioxidant vitamins A, C, and E. The seaweed known as bladderwrack is one of several herbs noted for specific thyroid support. Most of these vitamins and minerals help transform L-tyrosine into thyroid and adrenal hormones. Low thyroid function is often reflective of poor general nutrition.

#18
Fat Blockers,
Fat & Sugar Substitutes

A natural way to reduce fat and sugar absorption by the body is to increase the consumption of fiber, especially from vegetables. Commercial sugar substitutes which provide the sweet flavor without the calories have been around for a long time. New products have now appeared which work specifically to reduce the absorption of fat or to replace the fats usually found in foods. In the first category the primary products are made from a type of fiber called chitosan, which directly binds fats before they can be absorbed and a protein fraction (a peptide) which both binds to fats and increases their clearance from the digestive tract. In the second category is the product Olestra. All of these approaches to reducing caloric intake claim to help dieters.

Chitosan is an extract form the hard outer shells of shellfish. These shells are their exoskeletons. In Japan this type of material was developed for use in water purification and other similar purification purposes, such as in the food industry. The principle is that there is a positive electrical charge on the chitosan which draws oppositely charged marterials to it. The same type of fiber was developed in Europe, and the principle of electrical charge was recognized as having a bearing on fat absorption. Fats and bile acids are negatively charged, and therefore are attracted to the chitosan and bound before they can enter the blood stream. The makers of chitosan products claim that fats equal to seven to eight times the weight of the chitosan can be blocked in this fashion.

A quite different approach to absorbing and trapping fats uses components found in certain proteins. This protein "globin digest," is prepared by a special acidic protease (protein digesting) treatment. Peptide FM is the marketing name for the small chain of peptides which makes up globin digest. A combination of bovine (cow), milk and/or wheat proteins provide the starting materials. The claim is that the digestion, aborption and metabolism of fats are regulated by this material. Non-digestible sugar substitutes, whether sugar alcohols or specially alterred amino acids, such as make up Aspartame (NutraSweet™), which are used, for instance, to sweeten diet drinks, have been around long enough to become part of billion dollar industries. If *faux* sugar, why not *faux* fat? Olestra is the new "fat-free fat" marketed by Proctor & Gamble and developed at a cost reputed to be well above $200 million. The basic principle is simple. Regular fat consists of fatty acids arranged around a type of alcohol called *glycerol*. In the digestive tract various enzymes cut through the links which bind the fatty acids to the glycerol to create units small enough to pass through the intestinal wall and into the blood. Olestra, however, has a very large center made of the sugar sucrose instead of glycerol, and around this center are arranged six to eight fatty acids. The result is a molecule which is much bigger than normal fats and which has fatty acids so tightly packed together that digestive enzymes cannot reach the crucial links to snip off the fatty acid components. The olestra molecule itself is too massive to pass through the intestinal wall.

How Do They Work?

Chitosan has been tested more than once against the FDA-approved drug Questran (*cholestyramine*). Questran removes bile acids from the liver and effectively lowers cholesterol levels. Chitosan binds liver bile acids, but it primarily binds dietary cholesterol and other fats. In head-to-head tests, the drug was more effective in lowering cholesterol, yet the researchers were able to conclude that "chitosan may have lipid-lowering effects similar to those of cholestyramine..." Chitosan is used to reduce the absorption of fat from the diet. In effect, it is intended to allow the dieter to follow a low-fat diet without cutting fat from the diet.

The results reported by the European supplier of chitosan were twice the weight loss found with the controls during the first two weeks and roughly another 5 pounds better weight loss over the next two weeks. Blood pressure lowering effects were also significant. Compared to Questran, chitosan is certainly safe.[77] Nevertheless, some researchers have questioned the wisdom of the long-term use of chitosan.

The original use of this type of fiber in Japan was to clear metals from water, and, as this implies, chitosan may bind minerals found in the diet as well as fats. Similarly, fat soluble vitamins and other such nutrients are unlikely to be distinguished from cholesterol by chitosan, and therefore a deficiency in vitamins such as A and E and in nutrients such as beta-carotene might develop. Japanese researchers have actually performed experiments with animals to see if chitosan taken in large amounts will have a negative effect on the mineral and vitamin status of the body. Their findings were that mineral absorption was greatly decreased, the bones were demineralized and that there was a "marked and rapid decrease in the serum vitamin E level...."[78]

Peptide FM in several unpublished studies was shown to decrease total body fat and serum triglycerides in humans as well as in animals. Over a three month period, body fat levels typically were reduced about 3% with no other changes in diet or exercise. The explanation for these results offered by researchers is that movement of fat into the bloodstream from ingested food is reduced and that the overall turnover of fats by the body, including oxidation for energy, is increased.[79] A further claim that the synthesis of new fat from carbohydrates is reduced is probably an indirect effect due to the improved insulin response usually found when there is better clearance of free fatty acids from the blood. No side effects have been reported.

Olestra, the non-fat fat, is included here because soon it will be found routinely in the food chain, from chips 'n dips to ice cream and beyond. It works by simply replacing fats in the diet with a non-digestible sucrose polymer. Unfortunately, various researchers, including those who testified before the FDA, have noted that Olestra binds and removes fat-soluble nutrients from the body. These include carotenes, vitamins A, D, F, and K. Olestra also apparently causes diarrhea in some individuals.[80]

An interesting secondary issue is whether these caloric-free sweeteners and fats succeed in helping dieters to lose weight. More than one bariatrician has told the author that dieters who do not lose weight when treated medically typically are those who drink the largest amounts of sugar-free diet drinks. This curious result could come from the amount of sodium found in those drinks, which might encourage water retention in some individuals, or other factors might be involved. Saccharin may in fact help slightly with weight loss under some conditions, but aspartame appears to downregulate the enzyme responsible for thermogenesis by as much as 30%! In either case, however, the mere use of artificial sweeteners may lead to greatly increased fat consumption when compared to a similar use of sugar. Similarly, one study found that when subjects consumed artificially sweetened drinks during exercise, they ate 160-190 more calories from all sources at lunch than did individuals who drank plain water or a sucrose flavored drink![81]

One likely explanation is that the mere "sweet taste" on the tongue may stimulate the release of insulin. Research on this point has been equivocal for the moderate consumption of "sweet taste," (which does not rule out the suggestion). In contrast, it does seem to be clearly proven that the consumption of "sham" food which taste like the real thing, but which has no calories, leads to significant elevations of blood insulin levels. When Olestra was used to replace fat calories in a restricted-calorie diet, a recent study found that dieters simply ate more calories to make up for the lost fat calories if given access to more food.(6) *The implication is that the consumption of the new reduced-calorie imitation foods will not help dieters either take off or keep off weight.*

Availablility and Dosage

Chitosan is taken in amounts which vary to match the fat content of a meal. It is available in tablets and capsules. Directions will come with products, e.g., one slice of pizza with 20 grams of fat might be balanced with 10 chitosan capsules. Peptide FM will usually be found as a component in diet powders and similar products. The amount recommended to control the fat in an average diet is from 1.5 grams to 2 grams.[82]

#19
CLA

Anti-Fat Nutrient	Conjugated Linoleic Acid.
Fat Burning Function	Regulates Fat Accumulation and Retention.
Suggested Dose	1,000-2,000 mg in divided doses with meals.

CLA (Conjugated Linoleic Acid)
In Depth

What Is It?

Conjugated linoleic acid (CLA) is a fatty acid nutrient which occurs naturally in beef, turkey and many dairy products. It was discovered in the mid-1980s by researchers who found that a compound in beef exerted an anti-cancer effect. Further investigations indicated that CLA is an immune system modulator — it alters some immune functions and how the body reacts to immune stimulation. As a rule, activation of the immune system can lead to the loss of lean tissue, but animals fed CLA did not suffer from wasting and other adverse effects to the same extent when injected with toxins or certain types of vaccinations.[83]

Currently, scientists believe that CLA alters the way that fats are broken down and stored in various membranes and tissues. The ratio of saturated fats to monosaturated fats in tissues is increased. The effect of this change in the several species of animals studies is a reduction in food consumption, a reduction in stored fat, a better ratio of high density lipoprotein cholesterol (HDL, the "good" cholesterol) to low density lipoprotein (LDL) and total cholesterol, and a reduction in atherosclerosis.[84]

CLA was originally available from animal fats. Currently, CLA is produced commercially from sunflower oil.

How CLA Can Help You Lose Fat

CLA has shown its best results as a protective agent against cancers and as a modulator of immune function. Under challenging conditions, CLA prevents the catabolism (tissue breakdown) which accompanies excessive immune stimulation. This may be important to dieters in that long-term stress is known to lead to weight gain. CLA also apparently changes to some extent the metabolism of lipoproteins (fats carried in protein packets) and the way in which the body utilizes fats for energy. In animal studies, CLA reduced overall food consumption and its use led to less weight from fat, although not necessarily to less total weight.

It should be pointed out that the results of these tests varied dramatically from species to species. Most of the studies done to date have focused on CLA's benefits in improving lean weight gain in animals eating less food.[85] No human studies have been conducted, and therefore the actual weight loss benefits at this point are speculative. From the results found with animals, it is likely that CLA may have some minor benefit in helping humans to stay or become somewhat leaner, but not necessarily lighter.

How Is It Available and How Should It Be Taken?

CLA has only recently become available at prices appropriate to a nutritional supplement. It is an oil which is supplied primarily in capsule form. Its makers usually recommend that 2,000 mg. of CLA be taken per day taken in divided doses, and it is likely that an effective daily dose must be at least 1,500 mg. per day.

CHAPTER 3

THE ANTI-FAT NUTRIENT
WEIGHT-LOSS PROGRAM

The core program involves the use of L-carnitine, the trace minerals chromium and vanadyl sulfate, fiber, spirulina, GLA and a lipotropic formula (see page 75). These nutrients are useful to those wishing to get leaner, control their appetite and improve their insulin regulation. The functions and uses of these nutritional supplements are discussed in detail in the previous section. To the core program you should add other nutrients which you think may be helpful to you. This list might include thermogenic aids (for faster weight-loss), lipogenesis inhibitors, and others. Probably everyone should take a good multi-vitiamin/mineral formula as well as extra antioxidants, such as vitamins C, E, and beta-carotene, and preferably also one or more of the flavonoids or other more recently discovered antioxidants discussed in Chapter Two. Lastly, dieters might try the simple, yet effective and satisfying diet described in Chapter Four.

For a large percentage of those who are over their ideal weights, the most important single supplement, really a food more than a supplement, is what is collectively known as the essential fatty acids (EFA's), especially the omega-6 fatty acid called gamma-linolenic acid (GLA), which is derived from linoleic acid (see GLA, Chapter 2). GLA affects the production of a whole series of hormones, and through these it plays a significant role in fat metabolism. Since so many of our modern processing techniques for oils and other foods seriously interfere with the body's use of GLA, this fatty acid, along with added fiber, constitutes an addition to the diet which can be recommended to virtually all overweight individuals.

Beyond these general suggestions, it must be pointed out once again that individuals gain weight for different reasons having to do with their metabolic individuality and the lives they lead. For instance, those who eat to control nervousness may be helped more by herbal relaxers than by any full scale frontal attack upon their waistlines (see the anti-stress nutrients to follow). Thermogenesis-inducing items, such as caffeine, may not be useful for those who are already prone to nervousness or for those who exhibit pituitary-related hypothyroidism, yet for those suffering from simple cases of dieting-induced sluggish metabolisms, such items may prove very effective.

Perhaps more important than the vitamins are the minerals, which should include calcium, chromium, copper, magnesium, manganese, potassium and zinc. These are especially important to dieters, but they are more broadly useful in controlling blood pressure and insulin response. Magnesium, zinc and the vitamins B-3, B-6 and C are necessary for the conversion of polyunsaturated fats in the diet into hormones. Magnesium and potassium are necessary for the activation of brown adipose tissue (BAT) for thermogenisis.

Two nutrients should be given a second look for other reasons. Vitamin B-6, which is easily destroyed in cooking of any sort, is important for protein metabolism and synthesis, and it has been shown to have an impact on some forms of diabetes.[86] Morever, it also has been demonstrated that men (more so than women) in their 60's rapidly can be made much less insulin sensitive (i.e., non-reactive to insulin) by being fed a diet lacking in B-6.[87] A chromium deficiency even more strongly is linked to blood sugar problems than is a deficiency in vitamin B-6. This mineral directly affects the body's response to insulin.

Indeed, one of the classic dysfunctions which appears with age and also with obesity is the reversal of the quantities of two antagonistic hormones produced by the body: insulin and growth hormone. On the one hand, insulin (which stores calories as fats and controls blood sugar levels) is produced in only small amounts when we are young, and we do not need much at that time since in youth our tissues are quite sensitive to insulin. On the other hand, human growth hormone (GH) is abundantly produced in the bodies of teenagers and young adults, and this is one of the reasons young people can "eat anything" and still not get fat. GH helps the body metabolize fat for energy by drawing the fat from its storage reserves.

Unfortunately, GH release gradually declines after the age of thirty. Excess fat storage itself upsets the body's hormonal balance and depresses the production of GH. As we age we also tend to produce more insulin because our tissues become less sensitive to its effects. One side effect of excessive insulin production and insulin tolerance is the tendency to put on weight. By adding the vitamins B-6, C and the mineral chromium to the diet we can better affect both the production of growth hormone and the regulation of insulin.

Results In Fifteen Days

Any well-designed nutrient-based diet program should be given 2 to 3 weeks to produce results. For instance, a well-designed thermogenic product which incorporates the herbs and supporting nutrients described in the previous chapter will work better the second week than during the first, and better the third week than during the second. The reason for this is that your body has a great deal of built in inertia or resistance to change. However, with the proper approach almost any dieter can expect to take off **and keep off** from 1 to 2 pounds per week during the first 3 weeks while actually improving energy levels and muscle tone. Give your chosen program at least 2 weeks to begin to deliver results and judge yourself by how you feel and by how you look rather than by numbers on the bathroom scale alone.

Fat-Burning Products

Numerous vitamin and pharmaceutical companies are now selling weight-control products based on the Anti-Fat Nutrients described in this book. These formulas are getting better all the time and now there are some quite effective fat burning products on the market. These products usually consist of multi-nutrient tablets which include some of the Anti-Fat Nutrients. Due to size limitations, it is difficult to include effective amounts of more than one Anti-Fat Nutrient category in such a tablet. For example, some products contain mostly lipotropics, whereas others provide primarily thermogenic nutrients. While you can obtain a measure of success by using just one special nutrient or category of nutrients, your results can be enhanced by using a variety of Anti-Fat Nutrients at the same time. Whether you choose to use one of these products, design your own program or use the program which follows, you should read about the nutrients in Chapter Two.

The following program is based on the experiences of the author as a nutritional consultant. A physician should be consulted before starting any nutrition or exercise program.

Before taking any of the following nutrients, please read Chapter Two for important additional information . See Chapter Two also for potencies of nutrients not mentioned below.

The Core Program

At least 30 minutes before Breakfast: 1 glass warm water with 3-6 spirulina tablets, 2-3 GLA capsules and 250-500 mg L-carnitine, 500 mg HCA.*

With Breakfast: A multi-vitamin/mineral supplement (can be taken with lunch instead), 200 mcg chromium, 5 mg vanadyl sulfate, antioxidants, a lipotropic formula, other augmenting nutrients.

Mid Morning: If taking a thermogenic product, take it at this time with a glass of water.

At least 30 minutes before Lunch: 1 glass of water, 3-6 spirulina tablets, 2-3 GLA capsules and 250-500 mg of L-carnitine, 500 mg HCA.

With Lunch: A multi-vitamin/mineral supplement (can be taken with breakfast instead), 200 mcg chromium, a lipotropic formula, antioxidants, other augmenting nutrients.

Mid Afternoon: If using a thermogenic product, take it at this time with a glass of water.

At least 30 minutes before Dinner : 1-2 glasses of water with 5-7 fiber capsules, 500 mg HCA.

With Dinner: 2-3 GLA capsules, a lipotropic formula, 5 mg vanadyl sulfate, anti-oxidants, other augmenting nutrients.

Note: It is important to drink extra water when taking fiber supplements.

* 500 mg of HCA is found in 1000 mg of a 50% HCA calcium salt or a 50% HCA potassium salt.

Augmenting Weight-Loss Nutrients

In Chapter Five we will see that false hunger can occur from low blood sugar, from stress and anxiety, from depression and boredom, and from nutrient deficiencies which come from eating refined food (which include white sugar, white flour products and white rice). The following nutrients can help each of these conditions.

Anti-Sugar Craving Nutrients: Adequate dietary protein, complex carbodydrates, chromium (minimum dose 400 mcg/day in divided doses) and vanadyl sulfate (5-15 mg/day). L-glutamine 500 mg-1 gm three times per day between meals may help.

Anti-Stress /Anxiety Nutrients: Magnesium, B vitamins, Vitamin C, DMAE, Pantothenic Acid, Valerian herb.

Anti-Depression Nutrients: L-phenylalanine, L-tyrosine, Gingko Biloba herb, Vitamin C.

Anti-Appetite Nutrients: Fiber capsules, spirulina tablets before meals, L-phenylalanine, L-tyrosine, thermogenic nutrients, and extra water. HCA reduces appetite but allow one to two weeks for the full effect to develop.

Also Consider:

• Additional antioxidant nutrients.

• Digestive aids.

• Thermogenic aids for those not suffering from nervousness or related conditions.

• Other supplements geared to body type, living habits and special circumstances.

For further information on special healing herbs and nutrients and for help in dealing with specific conditions, readers should consult one or more of the following:

Robert H. Garrison and Elizabeth Somer, *The Nutrition Desk Reference*, 2nd edition (Keats, 1990).

James F. Balach, M.D. and Phyllis A. Balach, *Prescription for Nutritional Healing* (Avery, 1990).

Simon Y. Mills, *Out of the Earth* (Viking, 1991).

Michael Murray and Joseph Pizzorno, *Encyclopedia of Natural Medicine* (Prima, 1991).

Ron Teeguarden, *Chinese Tonic Herbs* (Japan Publications, 1984).

Melvyn R. Werbach, M.D., *Healing Through Nutrition* (Harper Collins, 1993) and *Nutritonal Influences on Illness*(Keats, 1988).

CHAPTER 4

FOOD FACTORS

Anti-Fat Nutrients can help you lose weight without changing your diet or increasing your activity level. However, your results will be far greater if you include regular exercise and make important dietary modifications a part of your total weight control lifestyle. This section explores food and nutrition and offers some dietary practices which will make you feel great and facilitate healthy weight loss.

NUTRITION MADE EASY

Good nutrition is based on supplying yourself every day with more than forty essential nutrients. Throughout the ages this has been accomplished by the consumption of foods from the following food categories.

Animal Foods

1. Meats
2. Dairy
3. Eggs

Plant Foods

1. Grains
2. Vegetables, seaweeds
3. Beans and legumes
4. Nuts and Seeds
5. Fruits

Although it may be possible to receive all the nutrients you need from a limited food selection, it is more enjoyable, convenient and probably more healthful to include foods from all the food categories.

Go anywhere in the world and you will find cultures eating foods from all of the categories along with their favorite staple within each category. For example, people in the Western Hemisphere emphasize wheat within the grain category, whereas people in the Eastern Hemisphere emphasize rice. One good reason to consume a variety of foods is that a monotonous diet has been implicated in the development of food allergies.

After years of confusing and often contradictory nutritional information, there is now general agreement that the basic balanced diet should consist of foods high in complex carbohydrates and fiber, such as whole grains and vegetables, be moderate in proteins, and be lower in fats. An increase in the consumption of fresh fruits and especially vegetables and a reduction in salt and sugar intake are also recommended. Controversy continues with regard to the role of fats in the diet, and this issue is discussed at length in Chapter 5 and 6.

The Dieting Dilemma

Most diets fail because they depend primarily upon reducing the number of calories consumed. Yet research proves that **low calorie diets** are **not** the solution to lasting weight loss. Almost every dieter knows from experience that restricting calories very quickly reduces energy levels despite the initial weight loss common with low-calorie diets. On a daily diet of even 1,000 calories, the metabolism begins to slow down within 2 or 3 days. Your resting metabolism uses 75% of all the calories you burn in a given 24 hour period and is reduced between 10 and 20% on most low-calorie diets. Since your metabolism is designed to protect you against famine, your body will always defend itself against any large reduction in calories. Even starvation diets stop working after 2 to 3 weeks. **The dieter's dilemma is that with low-calorie diets you must cut calories to lose weight, yet cutting calories itself slows the calorie-burning process.**

The weight loss on low-calorie diets consists almost entirely of water, and the rapid weight loss of the first few weeks stops as one hits a "plateau." But this is only the beginning of the dieter's problems. After a low-calorie diet, the body's base metabolism, which is the amount of energy produced at rest, will remain depressed for several months. Then comes the "yo-yo" or rebound effect as the pounds return — with a vengeance! **Low-**

calorie diets promote fat storage, not fat burning.

Any adequate diet program shows you:

1. How to turn **off** your body's **fat storage** mechanism
2. How to turn **on** your body's **fat burning** mechanism
3. How to increase your lean body muscle tissue
4. How to increase your energy levels
5. How to reduce excess hunger and food cravings
6. How to keep the weight off and avoid the "yo-yo" dieting trap.

These goals can be accomplished by practicing a limited number of scientifically formulated principles. The principles of **food coupling** are designed specifically to balance and regulate the two major weight-controlling hormones of the body, *glucagon* and *insulin*. (See Chapter 5 for details.)

Principles For Weight Loss

<u>**PRINCIPLE #1:**</u> **Break the fat storage cycle by making the right food choices and by practicing proper "food coupling."**

Fat is a concentrated source of calories with about twice as many calories per gram (9 per gram) as are found in either carbohydrates or proteins. Fat-heavy meals lack bulk, so they make it easy to consume hundreds of calories without feeling full. Worse, **when fat is eaten at the same time as simple carbohydrates, both the fat and the carbohydrates are pushed into storage.** This is to say that stored fat increases, blood fat levels soar and the body's basic blood sugar control mechanism is damaged. **The "bad" coupling of fats with carbohydrates slows down your metabolism and causes you to gain weight.** To avoid weight gain, avoid all sugars and simple carbohydrates and especially avoid fat/carbohydrate couplings such as are found in fried foods, cakes and cookies, sweet rolls, candy bars and so on. Avoid all fruit juices since these are concentrated sources of sugar. Limit whole fruits to 2 servings per day. Emphasize whole grains, legumes, lean proteins and lightly cooked fresh vegetables. **Limit fats to 30% of your total calories.**

Protein/carbohydrate couplings also should be kept to a minimum. Most protein foods contain fat (e.g., most meats, eggs, milk). Moreover, research indicates that protein/carbohydrate combinations may reduce the body's ability to release growth hormone (GH), a major fat-burning hormone.

PRINCIPLE #2: **Turn on your metabolism naturally with the proper food choices. Burn stored fat for energy and for body heat.**

Some foods burn "hotter" than do others, i.e., they cause your body to expend more calories for heat, encourage activity and are not as readily stored. Proteins and complex carbohydrates are "hot" burners. They are not easily stored as fat and they tell your body it has plenty of fuel, so it is all right to go ahead and spend energy. This is part of the "thermic" or heat-producing effect of eating a meal, and it "turns on" your metabolism. **Couple lean proteins (fish, skinless chicken, lean beef or lamb, tofu) with a variety of non-starchy vegetables for especially energizing meals.** If a meal contains no concentrated carbohydrates (no breads, grains, potatoes, etc.), you need not be particularly concerned about its fat content. **Couple complex carbohydrates with vegetables (and perhaps a small amount of lean protein) for satisfying and more bulky meals.**

PRINCIPLE #3: **Exercise to increase your metabolic efficiency and to train your body to burn stored fat for energy.**

Exercise burns calories, but the greatest benefit comes after the exercise has ended. If you walk briskly for a mere 30 minutes per day, you will increase your calorie burning for the entire 24 hour period. Adding a moderate amount of upper body exercise or weight lifting will improve your energy expenditure even more by adding calorie-burning lean muscle tissue to your body. **For weight loss, plan on walking briskly for at least 30 minutes**

every day. This is best done either before or after breakfast. A walk early in the day while the body's temperature is still rising will invigorate you for the rest of the day. A second choice as a time for a walk is after your last meal of the day. Walking after meals is a particularly good practice for diabetics and for those genetically prone to developing diabetes.

PRINCIPLE #4: **Add fiber to your diet, especially in the form of lightly cooked green vegetables. Avoid refined and processed foods whenever possible.**

Fiber slows down food consumption so that your body has a chance to signal that you have eaten enough. It adds bulk to the meal to give you a feeling of satisfaction at having eaten. It slows the increase in the blood sugar level which follows any meal. Fiber carries waste products from the body and, especially if it comes from lightly cooked vegetables, it supplies important minerals and antioxidants. Try to vary your fiber sources. Avoid too much scratchy wheat bran, but add grains such as oats and barley and starchy vegetables such as sweet potatoes and yams (without added butter and sugar) to your menu. Try to eliminate refined and processed foods from your diet. Eliminate all canned and frozen foods — these often contain hidden fats and sugars.

PRINCIPLE #5: **Use anti-fat nutrients and thermogenic enhancers.**

Many individuals who are overweight find that they need a little help to "jump start" their ability to burn fat. See the basic program given in the previous chapter for guidance in designing your own anti-fat nutrient program.

TEN BASIC TIPS FOR WEIGHT LOSS

1. Drink 8-10 glasses of water every day. This will help your body rid itself of toxins and, surprisingly, it will also help you to reduce retained water. Limit salt and salty foods — these encourage water retention.

2. Never skip breakfast. If you skip breakfast, your body will take this as a sign that you are "starving" and slow down your metabolism. Substituting a cup of coffee and a sweet roll for breakfast is almost as bad as not eating that meal.

3. Chew food thoroughly. Do not eat in front of the TV or in other situations in which eating is "automatic" or unthinking.

4. Eat supper at least 3 hours before going to sleep. Eating late in the day causes food to be stored as fat rather than burned for energy. Eating late also makes it more difficult to wake up in the morning.

5. Eat moderate portions. Smaller meals digest better and keep energy levels more stable. Change snacking habits. For snacks at mid-morning or mid-afternoon, try raw vegetable slices, whole fruits or a cup of vegetable soup.

6. Eat one tablespoonful of cold/expeller pressed oil daily, preferably at a meal containing a lean protein. Choose from flax seed oil, walnut oil, canola oil, or safflower oil. These oils contain essential fatty acids which actually turn on your body's metabolism. These can be used as salad dressings and in sauces for vegetables, or even mixed into low-fat cottage cheese for a simple protein meal. **Do not cook these oils.** If you must saute a food, use olive oil.

7. Avoid caffeine unless it is specifically a part of your Anti-Fat Nutrient program. Caffeine in excess or taken late in the day prevents sound sleep. Sound sleep in the first few hours after going to bed is important for the proper functioning of the body's hormonal system.

8. Encourage maximum weight loss by having two protein-based meals and one carbohydrate-based meal per day according to the following coupling meal guide. For

maintenance and long-term health considerations, eat one protein-based and two carbohydrate-based meals per day.

9. Limit alcohol consumption to 2 glasses of wine or beer per day.

10. Do not become a scale watcher. Weigh yourself no more than once a week. Watch your mirror — you'll like what you see there!

FOOD COUPLING KEYS TO WEIGHT CONTROL

The Anti-Fat Nutrients Weight-Loss Program advocates a non-calorie restricted diet based upon a moderate and sustainable eating pattern. What you eat, when you eat it, and which foods you eat together are far more important than the number of calories you consume. Make informed food choices.

KEY #1: Avoid fat/simple carbohydrate combinations. Avoid all sugars. Eat no more than 2 servings of fruit a day and drink no fruit juices. Limit protein/carbohydrate combinations.

This is the most important part of your diet. Fat/carbohydrate combinations include all foods such as the following: French fries, buttered breads, cakes, cookies, candies, most bakery products, canned and frozen foods with added corn syrup or fructose, milk shakes, ice cream, most fast foods, packaged corn and potato chips, peanut butter sandwiches, most packages snack foods, etc. Simple sugars are found in fruit juices, soft drinks, most prepared breakfast cereals, many canned and frozen foods, and most so-called "diet powders" and "diet drinks." Eat unprocessed and unrefined foods whenever possible.

Small amounts of olive oil used in pasta sauces and in cooking are allowable.

KEY #2: Couple proteins with vegetables. Trim the visible fats from meats, but do **not** attempt to make protein meals "fat free." You can eat **unlimited** amounts of non-starchy (primarily green) vegetables and **limited** amounts of starchy vegetables at protein-containing meals. Small amounts (1/4 cup) of all nuts (raw) except peanuts can be eaten.

Proteins include, in order of preference, fish, turkey, chicken, other poultry, lamb, beef, pork, eggs and cheese. Beans/legumes are better considered as complex carbohydrates than as proteins. Milk interferes with the digestion of other proteins and should be taken alone. Unrestricted vegetables, which are best lightly steamed but may be sauteed in a little olive oil, include asparagus, green beans, broccoli, cabbage, cauliflower, celery, celantro, mustard and other "greens," green and red peppers, scallions, spinach and zucchini. Starchy vegetables, which should be limited to 1/2 cup at any meal containing fats, include beets, carrots, corn, green peas, pumpkin, and winter squashes.

KEY #3: Couple complex carbohydrates/starches with vegetables. Avoid fats and limit protein (less than 1/4 cup) at carbohydrate-containing meals. Small amounts (1/4 cup) of all nuts (raw) except peanuts can be eaten. Try to use natural insulin potentiating spices, such as bay leaf or curry, at meals which include rice or potatoes.

Complex carbohydrates include whole grain wheat, corn, barley, oats, millet, brown rice, buckwheat, amaranth, quiona. Excellent non-grain starches are potatoes, sweet potatoes, yams and most beans/legumes. These can be eaten in moderate quantities and vegetables can be eaten in unlimited quantities at these meals. Small amounts of olive oil used in pasta sauces and in cooking are allowable.

FOOD COUPLINGS FOR WEIGHT LOSS

DO'S	DON'T'S
FAT BURNING COUPLINGS	FAT STORING COUPLINGS

protein (4-6 oz.)+ green vegetables (limit starchy vegetables to 1/2 cup)	**protein + carbohydrates**
*carbohydrates + **all vegetables	**fats + carbohydrates**
*starches + **all vegetables	**fats + starches**
*carbohydrates + ***fruits	**proteins/fats + fruits**

*Complex carbohydrates/starches: whole grains, whole wheat pastas and breads, beans and legumes, potatoes, sweet potatoes and yams.

**Includes starchy and high carbohydrate vegetables: corn, beets, green peas, lima beans, snow peas and winter squashes.

***Exclude melons: Melons should be eaten alone.

Example Menus:

Protein-Based Breakfast: Cheese omelette, Spanish tomatoes and peppers, beverage.

Carbohydrate-Based Lunch: Baked potato, peas & pearl onions in curry sauce, corn and red bell peppers, 1/2 cup raspberries, beverage.

Protein-Based Dinner: Chicken breast, vegetable soup, sauteed pea pods with mushrooms, asparagus, salad (walnut oil & vinegar), sugar free sherbert, beverage.

The above menu gives good results for most dieters. However, dieters making use of HCA products such as CitriMax™ may find it advantageous to consume a slightly higher amount of complex carbohydrate. This is because HCA primarily influences carbohydrate and glycogen metabolism in suppressing the appetite. Other recommendations with HCA use include limiting intake of fat and alcohol.

CHAPTER 5

THE END OF DIETING

We all know famous personalities, such as Oprah Winfrey, who heroically and publicly have lost a great deal of weight on this or that special diet, only to regain the lost pounds month by month. Recently the National Institute of Health estimated that nearly 90% of dieters regain all or most of their lost weight within five years, then repeat the cycle of diet and weight gain once again. A large and thriving industry which sells billions of dollars a year in diet products and services, has grown up to take advantage of the difficulties and the frustration which many face when they attempt to lose weight. The aim of this book is to help its readers avoid both the desperation and the relapse so typical of dieting, and to do so without costing the hundreds of dollars charged by various special programs and clinics.

Any number of dieters have found themselves caught in this trap of using a crash diet to lose weight, only to have the pounds return with a vengeance and refuse to come off a second time. Others have lost weight, seemingly successfully, yet when they looked in the mirror they still did not like what they saw. There are at least five reasons for these sad results of good intentions and considerable effort. Three of these reasons are physiological and two are psychological, but quite real. To begin with the physiological issues, these include diet-induced hypothyroidism (low thyroid function) and other diet-induced metabolic imbalances, the loss of lean tissues and the ramifications of metabolic individuality.

Why Diets Don't Work Part 1

The physiological reasons apply to pretty much everyone who diets, and virtually no professional in the field of weight loss doubts their effects. As a general rule, diets which take off more than two pounds per week remove primarily water and/or lean tissue from the body. Diets based on diuretics ("water pills") do this directly, but much the same effect is achieved by most (but not all) low carbohydrate diets. For example, many high protein diets often work for a period of time because protein is an inefficient source of energy which floods the blood stream with nitrogen by-products as it is broken down to yield calories. Ammonia and urea are toxic to the body. They are known to be hard on the liver and even harder on the kidneys. Needless to say, these waste products do not make the dieter feel better. People lose weight rapidly on low carbohydrate diets mostly due to a loss of water as the kidneys draw moisture from the tissues in order to flush protein waste products from the body. This is to say that your body chooses the lesser of evils. However, as soon as the diet ends, the desiccated tissues are quickly rehydrated and the "lost" weight is regained.

Diets which are extremely low in calories—no matter how well balanced in terms of quality proteins, vitamins, electrolytes, and so forth—ultimately are counter-productive because they convince the body that it is starving, so it shuts down to conserve energy. The abrupt restriction of calories leads to diminished thyroid activity within as few as two days. This fact is significant because one of the main stimulants of energy consumption and of general physical activity is the thyroid hormone. The thyroid also is very important for *thermogenesis*, the production of body heat, and dieters usually should be aiming at increasing this process. Yet to guard against the seeming starvation of crash diets, the body shuts down thyroid production to conserve energy, and depression of thyroid activity in turn is linked to the reduction of fat mobilization and to an increase in fat storage. The results are that the dieter feels tired and that the number of calories burned daily actually declines. Similarly, since the body is trying to prevent starvation, it begins to use up not primarily the fat which the dieter wants to lose, but those tissues which burn calories, that is, the body's lean muscle tissues. The body's logic is simple: reduce the calorie-burning lean tissues and you reduce the danger of starvation. If this were not bad enough, the energy inefficiency and the sheer toxicity of many diets through yet other mechanisms again may cause the loss of lean tissues, including those of the heart.

To be sure, there are specially designed very low calorie/high protein diets which aim at sparing the lean tissues while encouraging moderate *ketosis*, the burning of the body's fat stores for fuel, but even the best of such diets run up against the body's defense mechanisms intended to prevent starvation. Moreover, since dieters can achieve the same mild ketosis of very low carbohydrate/high protein diets without expensive diet powders or liquids and without an extreme restriction of calories, the usefulness of even the best of the very low calorie/high protein diets is questionable. This is not to say that well-designed protein-sparing very low calorie diets cannot work to help one lose weight *in the short term*—clinically they often have been shown to lead to significant weight loss—but only to warn that they may not be the best way to go and that the weight lost through such diets will likely come back.

In brief, the body during a crash diet defends itself against what it perceives as starvation by cannibalizing the muscle tissue which uses up calories and thus threatens survival under famine conditions. At the same time the depression of thyroid production makes it harder for the body to burn fats. Indeed, as much as 30% of the weight lost during a typical crash diet is from muscle loss. Moreover, energy conservation measures can be so effective that some people cannot lose weight even consuming only 750 calories a day, which is about one third of a normal daily consumption of calories![88]

Weight Loss Is Easy — Fat Loss Is Not

Now for some slightly more technical explanations of what happens on crash diets. The first physiological change brought on by a crash diet is the loss of lean tissue, and this loss means that the dieter's entire metabolism slows down. Lean tissue burns calories 24 hours a day, and it is the muscle-to-fat ratio which often is most important in determining how well the body handles calories. The loss of lean tissue results in the lasting reduction of what is called the basal metabolic rate, the rate at which the resting body normally uses energy, whereas an increase in the muscle-to-fat ratio heightens the basal metabolic rate.[89] Therefore, after the crash diet ends, the body needs fewer calories to sustain itself, and even on a restricted maintenance diet the pounds will slowly return. Likewise, dieters may find that they seem to have permanently lost a certain amount of energy and perhaps, as well, that they do not respond properly to colder temperatures by increasing body warmth. And, of course, fat reserves, which do not burn calories, actually have become a larger proportion of all the body's tissues. When the disappointed dieters go back on their former diet, they find it much harder to lose the weight a second time since their metabolism has slowed down. The weight comes back more quickly, and often they gain even more weight.[90]

The second physiological change caused by crash diets is a bit more subtle than the first, but every bit as detrimental. When the body is presented with what seems to be starvation, it activates a number of hormones involved in fat storage while reducing the production of hormones which cause the body to burn fat for energy. The reduction in catabolic thyroid activity has already been mentioned. Other hormones, such as *insulin* and a liver enzyme called *lipoprotein lipase*, are anabolic in nature. Together these anabolic hormones and changes cause the body to begin to store food as fat, even when only a very few calories are consumed. (See the section later titled "Hypothyroidism, Liver Function and Brown Fat.") Once hormones such as lipoprotein lipase have been activated for any length of time under quasi-famine conditions, it is very hard to convince the body to turn them off again. Moreover, fat storage may begin even before the diet actually has ended. On some high protein diets the body can turn the excess protein into enough sugar so that the unused portion is stored by insulin as fat. As the dieter returns to a normal number of calories after the diet, the anabolic hormones continue to conserve energy and to store calories. After the diet is over, the unfortunate dieter may put on 10 pounds before the regulatory mechanisms quiet and return to something approaching their normal ranges. With successive crash diets, the body finds it easier to turn on energy-sparing hormones and more difficult to turn them off.[91]

A third physiological limitation of most diets is that they fail to take into account metabolic individuality and therefore they usually fail to address the actual causes of unwanted weight gain. Some people gain weight because they are inactive, some because of the combinations of foods in their diets, still others because of faulty regulatory mechanisms. It is highly unlikely that all these different individuals can be helped by using exactly the same diet, and the sources of their problems are not the same. (See the discussion below of body types.)

Aside from the severe physiological drawbacks of the usual crash diets, there are psychological drawbacks as well. For one, the dieter wants fat loss, not just weight loss. To get the proper "look," the desired shapeliness of the body, the body's fat must be where it belongs, that is, mainly between the skin and the muscle. Excess fat commonly is spread into other tissues. When this fat is lost, and much muscle along with it, although she or he may now be at the weight given as ideal on the charts, the dieter still looks and feels flabby. The diet has done nothing to improve the tone of the muscles or the shape of the body. As a result, the dieter feels unsatisfied even after having lost a great deal of weight.

A second psychological drawback of most diets is that they do not address the cravings which cause many people to overeat or to eat the wrong foods. These cravings themselves often have a basis in physiology or even in brain biochemistry, so they seldom are "all in one's head." But regardless of how the cravings are defined, a brief look at a few of them will show why diets rarely are the answer to the mischief such cravings cause. Surveys have shown that half of all respondents admit that they tend to use food as an answer to depression. Significantly, solace is not sought in protein foods, for which consumption remains largely steady under a variety of circumstances, but in fats, sweets and other carbohydrates. In one poll done for the *Wall Street Journal*, ice cream and chocolate bars topped the list of mood-dependent food choices, followed in order by pizza, beer, soft drinks, hot soup, peanut butter and hamburgers.

Sometimes cravings are rooted in memories of home or happy times; sometimes they are rooted in desires to be "bad" or to punish oneself or others. Yet brain chemistry may supply better answers than simple memory. Judith Wurtman, a nutritional chemist at MIT, argues that carbohydrates tend to calm us and to provide energy while relieving depression. Reactions vary with individuals, but the calming response appears to be related to the ability of carbohydrates to increase the presence of the neurotransmitter serotonin in the brain while at the same time the increase in blood sugar temporarily elevates mood in those with uneven blood sugar control. (Proteins, in contrast to carbohydrates, tend to stimulate the central nervous system and thus make us more active.)

Adam Drewnowski of the University of Michigan suggests that the neurochemical link may be even stronger. Food cravings in some people may alter the level of endorphins, naturally occurring potent mood-altering brain chemicals which are similar to narcotics in their effects. Drewnowski's research indicates that many food cravings can be blocked by the drug naloxone, which in clinical settings sometimes is employed to ease opiate cravings.[92]

The point is that most diets attempt to reduce only the consequences of food cravings when such cravings lead to excess weight. These diets do nothing to reduce the cravings themselves nor to address their causes. Thus, just as these diets fail for physiological reasons to keep weight off (i.e., they do not prevent the "yo-yo" vicious circle of weight loss-weight gain) these diets also fail to address the many aesthetic and psychological aspects of weight loss and gain. (Specific diets are discussed in the section "Why Diets Don't Work Part 2.")

Your Ideal Weight

Before beginning any program for personal transformation, it is a good idea to consider why this change is desirable and just what it is that you want to achieve. Losing weight is no exception to this rule. Good reasons include considerations such as health, beauty and athletic performance. Bad reasons often mimic good reasons, but usually bad reasons can be recognized as involving unrealistic expectations and other psychological reasons rather than in one's physiology. One of the most common unrealistic expectations concerns appearance. TV and the press bombard us with images of "ideal" bodies, images of models and athletes, and so forth, but these are images which represent the natural body types of only a small percentage of the population—they are not most of us. Finding one's ideal weight means finding a healthful and sustainable weight which fits one's own metabolic individuality.

METABOLIC BODY TYPES AND FAT METABOLISM

Physiologists commonly divide all of us into three general body types, those of ectomorphs, mesomorphs and endomorphs. These body types are inherited, although they can be influenced by diet and activities during the first two decades of life. Body types are rough guides to individual metabolic rates and to fat metabolism. It is not possible for us to change our body types, and therefore it is unrealistic to expect any program of diet or exercise to accomplish this feat. Dieters should discover what is realistic for their own body types and likewise discover the strengths which are the special virtues of each type. This is a much better approach than for all of us to attempt to be the same "ideal" person.

For instance, the *ectomorphs* are naturally slender individuals who find it difficult to gain weight no matter how much they eat. Their metabolisms are fast burning and their ability to convert food to fat is limited. Often they have great difficulty in putting on muscle tissue as well. These "thin no matter how much they eat" types are often the envy of their heavier cousins, but this attitude is very much a product of the plenty which characterizes food sources for most Americans. Historically, the ability to gain weight when food was plentiful was a survival mechanism. It defended against periods of famine and it insulated the body against cold. These facts can be seen geographically in the populations of Europe. There is a crude gradient which runs from the warmer and more temperate West and South (e.g., England, France and Spain) to the generally colder East (Russia). Naturally occurring body fat is a higher percentage of total body weight in the East than in the West, and this inherited physiology reflects in part the harsher climate and the more unstable food supply as one moves eastward. Being an ectomorph may be great if you want to be a basketball star or a willowy fashion model, but it is not so good if you want to survive a winter in Siberia.

Can ectomorphs become obese? Yes, they certainly can. Typical ectomorphic cases of obesity may have been pencil thin in their early twenties or even later, but then they begin to gain weight rapidly. Ectomorphs are more prone than are other body types to psychological factors, such as nervousness, worry, anxiety and fear. To calm their nerves they may overeat and, especially, they may indulge in sugars and simple carbohydrates since these foods tend to encourage the production of the calming neurochemical serotonin in the brain. Also, feelings of security or stability may come with the added weight. For these nervous types, calorie restriction is likely not the primary answer to weight problems. Rather, calming the excess nervousness, whatever its source, is the better solution. Whole grains and starchy vegetables can help calm the nerves without encouraging excess pounds, and various herbs and moderate exercise can be tried to reduce hyperactivity. This body type will also benefit from regular schedules for activities and meals.

Mesomorphs are your typical athletic types. They tend to be large-boned, more heavily muscled and lean in their earlier years. Many of our champion bodybuilders are of this type, as, again, are many fashion models and actresses. Arnold Schwarzenegger and

Jane Fonda come immediately to mind. Gifted with physical prowess in their early and middle years, mesomorphs are likely to begin to put on weight in later life as they slow down metabolically (we all do) and cease to be as active, yet continue to eat much the same diet as they had in their youth because they have much the same appetite. Some of those most dissatisfied with their bodies after, say, age 40, are mesomorphs.

Weight gain in mesomorphs is most commonly the result of simple overconsumption. The appetite is good, so eating is satisfying in itself. The weight gained by mesomorphs often is much "firmer" than is that gained by ectomorphs, for the mesomorphs continue to have more muscle. Mesomorphs also like the feeling of power and stimulation given to them by red meats and other concentrated proteins, and also by spicy and fatty dishes which activate the liver. However, in the usual American cuisine, red meats contain lots of fats as well as proteins, and all these dishes are often combined with one or more relatively simple carbohydrate. Such combinations tend to have highly undesirable effects upon insulin production, and this leads to fat storage. Finally, in as much as excess protein intake makes most people more aggressive, mesomorphs, who do not usually need any additional drive or aggression, tend to consume beer and other alcoholic beverages "to relax." Alcohol itself has many calories and it also interferes with the metabolism of fat. Neither of these qualities is useful for someone who is overweight.

As a rule, of our three body types, it is the mesomorphs who can most easily regain their proper proportions simply by reining in the consumption of excess calories *if their weight gain has not gone on for too long and/or become too excessive.* True obesity, the gain of weight to something above 20% of one's ideal weight, tends to strongly derange the metabolism. Whether this is ascribed to the body's having established a new "set point" (either a brain or a fat cell-mediated level of body weight) or to other mechanisms, once the derangement has taken place, it requires considerable effort to correct.

Endomorphs are the third body type. These individuals put on weight easily and do not shed it readily. They likely have been what they consider "heavy" for most of their lives. If not too excessively self-conscious about their weight, these individuals tend to be somewhat more relaxed and calm than the first two types. If their weight is brought into a balance appropriate for their body type, these individuals also tend to have considerable physical endurance and mental staying power. Famous opera singers notoriously have endomorphic characteristics, but so did the great philosophers St. Thomas Aquinas and David Hume. Many professional football players display large degrees of endomorphy, but so does Marlon Brando. And what woman is not envious of the hair, eyes and complexion of Elizabeth Taylor, who, again, has some strong endomorphic traits?

Endomorphic obesity often is related to a slow metabolism. This may be the result of inadequate thyroid production or of other hormonal conditions, it may be the result of the simple tendency toward inactivity or it may be the consequence of the desire to have comfort, such as good food. The kidneys may be slow and there may be a tendency toward water retention for any number of reasons. In any event, this body type does well by avoiding all simple carbohydrates and also excess salt. Since there is already a tendency to store excess calories as fats, endomorphs do well to restrict all sources of concentrated calories. Bulky foods, such as raw and cooked vegetables, whole grains and beans, etc., are good choices, as are foods which increase thermogenesis. Aerobic exercise to speed up the metabolism is a great idea; excess sleep and naps probably should be avoided. More especially, the amount of time spent in front of the television should be strictly controlled. TV watching has been shown to dramatically lower basal metabolic rates for many individuals, and the amount of time spent in front of the television is the second best predictor of obesity known![93]

These three body types respond differently to the same diets, and even at their ideal weights they will never look the same. And why should they? Most of us have bodies which are combinations of ectomorphy, mesomorphy and endomorphy in varying degrees. Each of us can obtain her or his own ideal weight, but it must match the body each of us has.

The ectomorph/mesomorph/endomorph taxonomy is a simple one commonly used, but it is not the only one available. Dr. Elliot D. Abravanel in the last decade wrote two books based upon the notion that each of us has a dominant hormonal system. During the same period Dr. Jeffrey Bland, a well-published author of books on nutrition, put his own candidate into the lists with a diet based upon the individual's efficiency at the metabolism of fats, carbohydrates and proteins. Yet another taxonomy, this one based upon the ancient Indian Ayurvedic medical system of classification and treatment, recently was published by Dr. Deepak Chopra. The interested reader might want to consult these authors for fuller treatments of the notion of individual body types.[94] Not surprisingly, there tends to be a large degree of overlap among the various systems used to classify physiological types. The suggestions given above are by no means definitive, but they are useful guides for where to begin for balancing one's own particular body type.

The usual medical definition of obesity includes anyone who is 20% over his or her desirable weight. This definition is tricky in that one's ideal weight depends upon the size and type of frame which characterizes the body. Large-boned individuals will quite naturally carry more weight than those with light bones, which is to say that ectomorphs and mesomorphs of the same age and height generally should not weigh the same. A number of charts and tables have been prepared listing desirable weights for men and women, and your family physician will likely be able to show you one or more of these. The most commonly used one was prepared for the Metropolitan Life Insurance Company in 1959. Those either far below or far above the listed weights are thought to be at considerable additional risk of various illnesses, and the 20% figure for medically defining obesity was derived from statistics which indicate that it is only at this point that the death rate begins to markedly exceed normal. That is, the mortality rate at this point climbs for those not *already* suffering from high blood pressure, high blood lipids and/or diabetes, all conditions which themselves are usually associated with excess weight. Some more cautious medical authorities define obesity as anything above 10% of one's desirable weight.

Another way of defining ideal weights is to use the percentage of adult weight which is devoted to fat. One source (*The Physician and Sports medicine,* April 1986) considers men obese if this percentage is above 25%, and women obese if it is above 30%. The body fat percentage associated with optimal health for men can range from 10-25%, and for women, from 18-30%.

Neither of these ways of determining ideal weight is without its critics, and there is little agreement over how much damage is inflicted on one's health by being *moderately* overweight. As with the case of body type variations, genetic background appears to be very important in determining just how much risk a few extra pounds pose to health. Discovering whether you qualify as obese under an accepted medical definition will probably require the help of a doctor.[95] In 1983 roughly 40 million Americans were estimated to be obese in the medical sense, and another 40 million were probably above their desirable weights; two thirds of these individuals were over the age of 40. There is a great deal of evidence that genetics plays a role in determining adult weight.[96] Nevertheless, it is likely that excess weight for most "heavy" individuals is the result of inadequate exercise and/or faulty diet or related reasons.

Since the majority of readers no doubt already are aware that obesity brings health risks, the point will not be belabored here. Virtually all those involved medically in the care of the overweight, no matter their other differences, agree on a long list of complaints either directly or indirectly linked to excess weight. This list includes most or all of the following: "increased risk of stroke, diabetes, high blood pressure...diseases of the heart, blood vessels, liver, kidneys, and gall bladder."[97] Fortunately, many of these conditions can be stabilized or even improved through the loss of excess weight.

This list of ailments is a bit frightening, and it should be. More disturbing, however, is the fact that dieting itself often greatly worsens a bad situation. Crash diets place extreme stress on the body. The rapid weight gain which usually follows fad diets is more damaging in that it causes the elevation of unwanted blood lipids, increased rates of deposit of plaques on artery walls, and other damage to the body. The Framingham Study of heart disease indicated that those who were obese at the start of the study and who lost 10% of their body weight cut their chances of heart disease some 20%, but if they gained back those same pounds their risk rate jumped 30%, that is, it became higher than it would have been had they never dieted.[98]

Nevertheless, the good news from the Framingham Study is that a 10% reduction of body weight for those who at the start were clinically obese is significant if maintained. Every extra pound above the ideal is associated with a 2% increase in mortality rates, primarily from heart disease and cancer.[99] Indeed, the weight/mortality connection is so strong that critics of American medical dietary recommendations for controlling blood cholesterol levels through changes in diet have often noted that unless the obese subjects lost weight, changing the composition of the diet to radically reduce saturated fat consumption generally had little or no significant effect on blood lipid levels, and certainly not on mortality rates.[100]

Your Ideal Weight

Your ideal weight, as already has been indicated, depends upon a number of factors. However, the two most important of these are the size and density of your bones, and the ratio of lean tissue to fat stores. Weight charts have difficulty in accurately placing individuals by bone weight, relying on visible features such as describing people as having small, medium and large frames.

Likewise, the ratio of lean to fat tissues is best measured medically by the displacement of water in a test of underwater weighing to yield the body's specific gravity. Often the first stage of weight gain involves no gain of weight at all, but rather the loss of muscle tissue and its displacement by adipose tissue. This shows up as a change in the specific gravity of the body. Only after the metabolism has begun to slow because of the loss of the energy-burning muscle does the individual begin to markedly put on weight and then find this weight difficult to remove. The moral is that scale weight taken by itself is less significant than is normally assumed.

Nevertheless, studies have shown that dieters are more successful by far in achieving a desirable weight and in maintaining that weight if they have an ideal weight clearly in mind. Therefore, readers might try this suggestion from *The Endocrine Control Diet*: "One rule of thumb that has been used for determining ideal body weight for men is 106 pounds for the first 5 feet of height and 6 pounds for each inch after 5 feet, plus or minus 10 percent according to frame size. The rule for women is 100 pounds for the first five feet, and 5 pounds per inch thereafter, with the same adjustment for frame size."[101] For the sake of comparison, consider that the so-called ideal weight for successful endurance runners has been estimated to be twice their height in inches, i.e., a male runner who is 5 feet 10 inches, or 70 inches tall, should weigh 140 pounds.[102]

Don't Count Calories

A calorie is a unit of energy, and technically, the "large" calorie used in nutrition is one thousand of the "small" calories used in physics. In the body calories are provided by the oxidation of food, a process which at bottom consists of the chemical reaction of carbon and hydrogen with oxygen to yield water and carbon dioxide. This oxidation supplies energy for movement, for warmth and to drive other chemical reactions. The usual stand taken in diet books and in the popular press is that calories consumed must equal calories burned, otherwise a person puts on weight. A pound of body fat is the rough equivalent of 3,500 stored calories, and supposedly eating only 100 excess calories a day will cause weight gain of about a pound a month. Just reversing the process is said to take off the added pounds.

If this presentation were all that there is to the body's use of calories, then the companies which make a mint selling scales, calorie charts of common foods and various prepared food items with their calories already counted should have succeeded long ago in putting an end to excess poundage in America. But there are still 70-80 million Americans who, despite in some cases considerable effort, have not been able to permanently lose unwanted weight. Why?

Part of the answer lies in the notion of metabolic individuality outlined above. It is not just the food eaten, but the nature of the person eating the food which matters. Restricting calories may work wonders for the individual who gained weight solely because of a bout of inactivity and excess consumption, but whose metabolism has not been otherwise altered by the excess. This is the case with some—not all—women who gain weight during pregnancy and need a little help afterwards in losing it. Yet for those genetically disposed toward weight gain, for those who have gained too much weight and kept it long enough to alter their body's regulatory mechanisms, and for those who for medical or other reasons have put on and kept on excess pounds, counting calories is usually a humiliating and futile exercise which does little or nothing to remove excess weight.

Energy requirements can vary 100% among individuals of the same age, sex and apparent body composition, and even those with the same relative amount of lean tissue can exhibit unexplained variations of 25%![103] Moreover, the body is not passive in the face of a changing supply of calories. It constantly modifies its own energy expenditures in ways which make nonsense of simple calorie in/calorie out equations. How can it be the case that the woman not losing weight on 750 calories a day is not restricting her food intake sufficiently?

Carbohydrates, Fats and Alcohol

As a rule, carbohydrates are the preferred source of energy. They burn the cleanest of all foods, producing only water and carbon dioxide as waste products. This means that carbohydrates place little burden upon the liver and kidneys. Carbohydrates likewise are the best source for the production of glycogen, a special sugar used and stored in the liver and in the muscles, and for the production of the blood sugar glucose needed by the brain. When carbohydrates are not available, the body breaks down protein—but not so readily fat—in order to supply the sugar necessary for brain function.

Fat supplies roughly twice the number of calories per gram (9 calories) as do either carbohydrates or protein (4 calories). Alcohol supplies 7 calories per gram. Although a certain amount of alcohol is routinely produced in the large intestine as a by-product of the action of bacteria and yeast and is readily detoxified by the liver, and although small amounts of consumed alcohol actually improve health, in quantities beyond a couple of beers or 2-3 glasses of wine, alcohol is toxic. Worse for the dieter, alcohol in any quantity inhibits the metabolism of fats, an action which itself involves the liver. Researchers reason that the liver must detoxify the alcohol before it can attend to the burning of fats, and this process slows fat metabolism by about a third.[104]

Fat may indeed have far more calories per gram than do other foods, but this does not mean that we can do without fats. There are a small number of polyunsaturated fats called *essential fatty acids* which the body cannot manufacture and which it cannot do without. Fats provide the basis for every hormone in the body and for essential components of all cell walls. Fats transport fat-soluble vitamins, such as A, D and beta-carotene. Fats constitute the sheaths of all nerves. Finally, lipids, i.e., fats, make up some 25% of the dry weight (the non-water weight) of brain tissue. As will be pointed out below, extremely low fat diets, when followed for long periods of time, appear to damage or exhaust important systems in the body. Extremely low fat diets (below 10% of all calories) have some recognized therapeutic uses, but they emphatically are not maintenance diets.

The Effects Of Excess Calories

Researchers in nutrition have shown that the results of the ingestion of a given number of calories depend upon many factors, the most important of which are probably the following:

a. the basal metabolic rate of the individual
b. the ratio of lean to fatty tissue of the individual
c. the degree and the duration of excess consumption
d. the amount of physical activity
e. the timing of food consumption, i.e., when eaten during the day and when eaten in relation to physical activity
f. the source(s) of the calories, i.e., whether protein, fat, etc.
g. the combination of sources of calories
h. genetic, disease or other unknown factors

Weighing these various factors properly can only be done on a case-by-case basis. However, there are some general rules which seldom are wrong.

First, it is possible for non-obese individuals with stable weights to modestly overconsume carbohydrates for periods of time without gaining weight. However, researchers generally agree that over long periods of time the consistent excess consumption of calories from carbohydrates (consumption of calories well beyond energy requirements) will lead to fat storage. The degree of response depends upon each subject's metabolic identity.

Second, for most individuals on mixed diets, that is, diets combining protein, carbohydrates and fats in the same diet, excessive amounts of fat are more likely to be stored as fat than are excessive amounts of carbohydrates. Reactions to mixed diets are greatly magnified, even distorted, when the carbohydrates are sugars or otherwise simple and refined in nature. See below for why this is the case.

Third, an excess consumption of carbohydrates is known to increase the body's production of lipogenic or fat storing enzymes, such as lipoprotein lipase.[105] The overfeeding of carbohydrates for long periods of time increases the body's ability to store calories as fat. Sugars are especially implicated in this process.

One form of sugar, *fructose*, the sugar found in fruit, is particularly noted for stimulating lipogenesis (fat storage). Fructose, unlike glucose, does not require insulin for its movement from the blood into the cells, and for this reason it is listed as being very low on the glycemic index (20), an index which rates the degree of blood sugar elevation triggered by foods in comparison with that triggered by glucose (100 on the index). This has fooled many into thinking that fructose is a sugar which can be eaten in large amounts—and, indeed, we Americans do eat it in large amounts since we consume large amounts of fruit, especially as juices. Also fructose makes up about half the sugar in corn syrups and in this form is added to most American processed foods, even many meats! Almost all of the fructose eaten is converted into glucose (causing a delayed insulin peak), and in animal experiments fructose elevated triglyceride and insulin levels so consistently that researchers concluded that fructose was more damaging than other sugars, not less. Fructose also increases blood uric acid levels, an effect which adds a burden to the kidneys and is involved in promoting gout.[106]

In general, the high sugar (e.g., sucrose, fructose, etc.) intake of the average American is implicated in chronic liver damage, fructose being perhaps the worst offender. Sugars cause significant increases in liver enzymes and, to repeat, the elevation of blood triglycerides. These findings suggest that the consumption of sugars can alter liver functions, perhaps permanently.[107]

Fourth, there is some evidence that the timing of meals is important. Calories eaten in the evening before bedtime are made available after the body has begun to slow down in preparation for sleep, and, hence are stored. Eating late in the day also inclines one toward skipping breakfast, and not eating a meal early in the day signals the body to conserve energy while leading to excess food consumption at the first meal eaten. Eating breakfast both warms the body, that is, in itself eating breakfast encourages thermogenesis, and signals the body that it is free to expend energy without fear of famine. Breakfast eaters tend to snack less and to consume less total fat. Eating the same total number of calories, obese subjects who ate three full meals have been shown to lose more weight than those who ate only lunch and supper.[108]

Fifth, getting regular exercise, in particular taking a short walk after meals, has many benefits. Moderate regular exercise (moderate here meaning merely 20 minutes 3 times per week) has been shown to aid in preventing obesity, heart disease, colectoral cancer and various psychological disorders.[109] Unfortunately, in the U.S. at the present time only 37% of individuals at the most physically active stage of their lives, students from the 9-12 grades, regularly get moderate exercise, a decline from 62% in 1984.[110] The good news, however, is that modifying the diet with the addition of moderate exercise really does work![111]

Exercise helps to control blood sugar levels without bringing insulin into play. Since insulin is one of the primary hormones involved in fat storage as it clears excess sugar from the blood, exercise, especially a mild form immediately after meals, for this reason alone would be worthwhile. Moderate exercise (aerobic only) also helps the body develop the ability to mobilize fat stores for energy. A brisk walk for 30 minutes twice a day raises the metabolic rate for a sustained period of time while helping to elevate the production of the enzymes which pull fat from storage. This process is called *lipolysis*, and it commonly is impaired in those who are overweight.[112] *Please note: It is not the calories specifically burned by the exercise during its brief duration which are most important!* The maintenance of lean tissues, the potentiation of insulin, the raising of the basal metabolic rate, etc., all continue long after exercise is discontinued. Considerable research shows that moderate exercise can significantly increase insulin sensitivity/glucose tolerance, and thus enabling the pancreas to produce less insulin.[113]

Dr. Grant Gwinup, Professor of Metabolism and Endocrinology at the University of California at Irvine, has rather neatly summed up the role of exercise in dieting as follows: "Exercising is far more effective than dieting in getting rid of excess weight. Individuals who diet without exercising lose mainly water and some muscle...When you're not eating enough food, when you're relying *only* on dieting to lose weight, your body fights back. It lowers your metabolic rate...However, if you exercise strenuously for 30 minutes or more daily, you will burn fat and keep muscle. You may not even have to cut down on food...Fat [also] is burned at a much faster rate."[114]

Sixth, increased consumption of dietary fiber, especially water soluble fiber, is helpful for improving health and reducing excess weight. The bulk of the fiber itself gives a physical feeling of fullness which helps to control how much is eaten at a given meal, and the high bulk and water content associated with fiber tends to slow down the process of eating to a point at which feedback signals of satiety from the brain can influence hunger/appetite and intestinal hormones similarly can be released which reduce food intake. Appetite is reduced directly by the bulk of the fiber and indirectly through the delayed emptying of the stomach and the release of hormones signaling satiety.[115]

Vegetable sources of fiber in particular usually combine few calories with large amounts of vitamins and minerals. There is considerable evidence that these micro-nutrients, especially minerals such as chromium, are necessary for proper insulin and lipid control. Meanwhile, the bulking action of soluble fiber slows down the release of carbohydrates into the blood from the intestines. The moderate rise in blood sugar levels associated with complex carbohydrates, especially with vegetables and legumes, likewise moderates the release of insulin into the blood and avoids the both the health dangers and the surges in appetite which characterize the body's responses to excessive insulin release.[116]

This last point brings up the issue of nutrition in general. A large amount of research suggests that the American diet, as a result of modern farming, storage techniques and food processing, is routinely deficient in the minerals responsible for blood sugar and lipid control. Other research indicates that the modern consumption of refined oils and the consumption of oils derived from the sources which we find to be most plentiful and cheap interferes with the body's mechanisms for fat storage and energy production. These issues are taken up in the next section and under the appropriate nutrients, such as GLA (gamma-linolenic acid.)

Finally, genetics plays a powerful role in contributing to obesity. This point was mentioned above under the discussion of body types, but it should be pointed out that there are specific genes which now are implicated in both obesity and diabetes. Interestingly, these genes find expression under similar circumstances, that is, with a diet such as that followed in the U.S., which is high in simple sugars, in fats and in total calories, yet low in physical activity. They control the production of the enzyme G6PD (glucose-6-phosphate dehydrogenase). This enzyme, as its name suggests, is a sugar storage enzyme which causes the conversion of sugar to fat for storage.[117]

THE USUAL CAUSE OF WEIGHT GAIN IN AMERICA

Dr. Scott Connelly, a highly respected expert in the field of nutrition, after reviewing numerous studies on diet and weight gain came to a conclusion which is of importance to anyone concerned about his or her weight. Connelly accepts that under conditions of excessive calorie consumption, dietary fat is more likely to contribute to body fat stores than is carbohydrate, but in his judgment this is not the primary conclusion to be drawn. Instead, he accepts that his review (like that of others) "demonstrates that even *small* amounts of mixed diet overfeeding will result mostly in fat storage, and lead to obesity if sustained for prolonged periods of time."[118]

In a nutshell, this means that eating too many calories on a regimen which mixes fats and carbohydrates will almost certainly lead to fat storage. *This should be amended to mean the consumption of fats in conjunction with simple carbohydrates in particular, for it is these carbohydrates which most markedly increase blood glucose levels and lead to derangements in insulin and lipid metabolism.* Historically in comparison with our own past, and in comparison with other well-fed populations which do not exhibit current American levels of obesity, this describes exactly the nature of our changed eating habits as Americans have become heavier and more prone to sugar and lipid-related disorders, such as heart disease and diabetes. For instance, already in 1962 Dr. Margaret A. Ohlson presented the following picture of changes in the American diet, a picture largely continued over the last 30 years:

Estimates of food available in retail channels per capita of population can be found in the reports of the U.S. Department of Commerce and, for recent years, the U.S. Department of Agriculture (for the period from 1889 to the present). Certain well marked trends can be identified. The consumer supplies of two basic sources of starch, i.e., cereals and potatoes, have decreased sharply. At the same time, the form of market cereals has changed from bread flour to highly processed bakery products and the prepared type of breakfast cereal. The per capita supply of refined sugar has increased from 50 pounds per person per year to about 100 pounds.[119]

The figure of per capita sugar consumption in the U.S. climbed until the 1980's with consumption peaking at about 120 pounds per year. Sugars of various derivations, e.g., fructose mentioned above, are now so commonly employed in hidden forms in almost all processed foods that keeping track of the actual figure has become very difficult. During this same period of time total fat consumption has remained largely stable, a small increase taking the form of more polyunsaturated fats, which have also become steadily a larger proportion of all fats consumed. Protein consumption by some estimates has actually declined slightly. Since an ever greater proportion of our food is processed in various ways, the amounts of various vitamins and minerals has declined absolutely. The addition of a few select vitamins and minerals after processing, and more recently the re-addition of fiber, is scarcely to be taken as an adequate return. The immediate link between carbohydrates and vitamins and minerals which is found in all traditional sources of food has been broken by many modern techniques of storage, handling and processing.[120]

The primary mechanism involved in weight gain on a mixed diet of fats and simple carbohydrates is that of insulin metabolism, and this data has been available since the 1930s. H.P. Himsworth early in that decade performed a number of dietary experiments in which subjects ate varying proportions of fat, protein and carbohydrate for a week or so before being given the then standard glucose tolerance test for diabetes. This test elevates blood sugar levels by the administration orally of a controlled amount of the simple sugar dextrose, after which the amount of sugar in the blood is sampled at 30, 60 and 120 minute intervals. The evidence showed that the higher the percentage of all calories in the diet which had been derived from fats in the interval before the test (usually a week), the higher the blood sugar levels after the administration of dextrose, i.e., the higher the level of glucose tolerance and the greater the impairment of response to the release of insulin.[121]

These findings have sometimes been taken as an indictment of high fat diets *per se*, but they actually prove exactly what they appear to prove, which is that sugars and other simple carbohydrates in the presence of fats cause an impaired insulin response. Fat metabolism uses different pathways than does carbohydrate metabolism, and the body cannot easily switch between the two, which is what the ingestion of simple carbohydrates—which now make up 40% of the American diet—demands. (The catabolic hormone glucagon, which mobilizes fat for energy and which also activates "brown fat," suppresses the anabolic hormone insulin, and vice versa.) An impaired insulin response allows large amounts of sugar to enter the blood without being controlled, something which results in the body's desperate release of far larger amounts of insulin. As more and more glucose enters the blood (too much is toxic), the body first turns this sugar into triglycerides (which make the blood thicker and "stickier") and then, via the now excessive amounts of insulin, these triglycerides are stored in fat cells. The presence of excess glucose in the blood itself interferes with the use of fat for energy and, through the action of the liver, again elevates the level of triglycerides and their storage as fat.[122] Fructose can be taken up in small amounts from the blood by the cells without the benefit of insulin. However, direct fructose metabolism is limited. Fructose can be fully eliminated from the blood only through the action of the liver, which converts fructose to glucose. The process of conversion merely delays the increase in the blood glucose levels, and it thereby delays the accompanying insulin spike. Significantly, a very large proportion of those who are overweight show signs of insulin resistance, and likewise, fully 80% of those who become diabetics as adults are overweight.[123] This indicates that the routine experience of highly elevated levels of insulin release damages the ability to respond to this hormone, and insulin resistance and obesity are linked together in the vast preponderance of cases.

Why Americans Are Fatter Than The French

The tendency toward a large percentage of the population carrying excess weight is a relatively recent phenomenon, and one much more characteristic of the U.S. than of Europe, as those who have traveled abroad can attest. For instance, the French in general show the diseases of excess and of age both less and at a later point of their lives than do their American counterparts; they are healthier and they live longer despite smoking far more. Why? They eat four times as much butter as we do, more than twice as much cheese which commonly is 60 or even 75% butterfat, and about the same number of calories. Indeed, the French eat more than twice the animal fats and only two thirds the supposedly healthful vegetable oils which Americans eat. *The French eat about half the whole milk and only one eighteenth— that is right, only 5.6%!—the sugar consumed in this country.* (We Americans, like the British, are notorious for our love of sugar.[124]) Frenchmen even eat only about one half the fruit which we consume, and therefore about one half the fructose from that source. (Since the French insist upon fresh foods, they avoid the fructose hidden in most processed foods.) On the other side of the ledger, the French consume more vegetables, more fish, more grains, more potatoes and more of other complex carbohydrates.[125] They also do not snack between meals, a habit which has been shown in overweight individuals to increase the total daily consumption of calories.

According to the advice of the popular press, the American food industry, the American Medical Association, and so forth, the French are doing just about everything wrong. According to the health statistics, they are doing something right, and that "something right" includes a diet with lots of fresh and whole/non-processed foods, but rather low amounts of sugars of any sort. They eat one-eighteenth the amount of refined sugar found in the American diet and about half the sugar from fruit, and that figure may well understate how much more sugar we Americans actually consume. If Dr. Connelly and others of like mind are correct, then it is the American diet, one simultaneously high in both fats and simple carbohydrates, which bears a large degree of responsibility for American weight problems.

(Lest the reader think that the French are the only exception, it should be pointed out that the Swiss, who are second only to the Japanese among industrialized countries in life expectancy, eat even more in the way of cheeses, butter and cream, sausages, etc. than do the French. No European group, however, appears to drink as much pasteurized and homogenized milk as Americans drink.)

If it is the American version of the mixed diet which is at fault for many of our health problems, including obesity, *then controlling the amount of fat in the diet is only one half of any solution.* To be sure, the higher the percentage of calories in the diet which comes from fat, the greater the degree of sensitivity to the negative effects of simple carbohydrates. However, as long as simple carbohydrates remain an important part of the daily menu, even the relatively small amounts of fats necessary for nerve health, the workings of the immune system, the processing of fat soluble vitamins, and so forth, will continue to pose a critical challenge to weight control. This realization, moreover, is not new, but quite old. For instance, the ancient Indians of the Asian subcontinent began the use of curry long ago because at least one of its chief ingredients, turmeric, controls excess reactions, i.e., an elevated insulin response, to the "sweetness" of white rice.[126]

Overall, the dietary problems of Americans can be rectified to a large extent merely by returning to the consumption of primarily unprocessed foods, including oils, and of unprocessed complex carbohydrates in general, by the movement to the occasional use of low glycemic index grains (e.g., more use of millet and barley, which in traditional medical systems are sometimes used to control diabetes, and less use of wheat and rice), by the reduction of the excessive consumption of fruit (especially as juice) and of any other sources of fructose, and by similar relatively minor dietary measures. To this regimen must be added a certain amount of moderate exercise to encourage the body to function properly. In those whose systems have already been damaged, a few more steps may be necessary to correct faulty fat metabolism, e.g., the addition of special essential fatty acids and other nutrients to daily foods.

HYPOTHYROIDISM, LIVER FUNCTION AND BROWN FAT

Hypothyroidism refers to the insufficient activity of the thyroid gland. Symptoms of this condition include extreme fatigue, memory loss, depression, nervousness, allergies, sleep disturbances, menstrual disturbances, reduced sex drive, digestive disorders and other problems. In as much as the thyroid hormone plays a major role in controlling the expenditure of energy, in the liberation and metabolism of stored fats, and in determining the basal metabolic rate, for the woman or man attempting to lose weight, the proper functioning of the thyroid is of considerable importance. Unfortunately, the refined diet characteristic of contemporary America tends to depress thyroid function.

The thyroid requires much more than just iodine to properly play its role in the body. Deficiencies of the vitamins A, B-2, C and E as well as of other nutrients long have been known to reduce the activity of this gland, and many authorities doubt that the current Recommended Daily Allowances (RDA's) of these vitamins are anywhere near adequate. Since low thyroid function is also correlated with excess blood lipid levels, it is clear that the various systems of the body are closely interrelated and that nutritional inadequacies affecting one system commonly spill over into and affect others. Those who are seriously overweight should have their basal body temperature and other indicators of thyroid function checked by a competent physician and make sure that they are consuming the nutrients important for thyroid function in adequate amounts.[127]

A second organ strongly linked to problems of fatigue and of sugar and fat metabolism is the liver. Liver dysfunction is found in a large percentage of overweight individuals,[128] and it was pointed out above that the consumption of refined sugars leads to liver damage. Rather unfortunately, hypothyroidism can worsen the effects of liver dysfunction in a direction which inclines sufferers toward the consumption of excess refined carbohydrates and weight gain.

It seems that in many cases of inadequate thyroid hormone secretion, the adrenal glands are influenced to reduce their own secretion of cortisol (hydrocortisone). Without the adrenal cortisol, the liver does not produce sufficient glycogen, its own special storage sugar also stored in the muscles, and this deficiency leads indirectly to hypoglycemia, that is, to low or to unstable blood sugar levels. This is much the same situation which arises with the excess release of insulin in response to the consumption of refined carbohydrates: the sufferer undergoes periods of extreme hunger despite the consumption of adequate numbers of calories.[129]

A special form of fatty or adipose tissue called brown fat makes up yet another aspect of the body's ability to regulate its energy consumption. Brown fat (brown adipose tissue or BAT) is common in infants, but its quantity declines as we age. Found in the neck, along the spine and arteries, and around the most important internal organs, this fat is "brown" because of the high concentration of mitochondria, which are cellular components designed to generate energy. Brown fat is the single most important engine for the body's production of heat, that is, for thermogenesis, whereas the fat under the skin, which is white because of its lack of mitochondria, functions primarily as insulation and storage.

This difference is decisive. In some people brown fat may make up as much as 10% of all fat, while in others it may be only 1 or 2%. At least part of this results from simple inheritance, and in animal studies it is clear that defective brown fat function can cause obesity.[130] However, diet, the environment and the degree of acquired heaviness all influence matters to a very large degree. For instance, in response to cold and to certain foods, the hypothalamus, a part of the brain which governs the sympathetic nervous system, releases the neurotransmitter *noradrenaline* (which also is called norepinephrine). Temperatures of about 72°F cause most fully clothed individuals to start to burn fat for heat. One of the drawbacks of obesity is its damping of normal thermogenic responses. Not only does sustained obesity alter the hormonal balance which controls lipolysis, such as the balance between glucagon and insulin, but the insulating qualities of subcutaneous fat blocks the dissipation of body heat, and thus turns off the thermogenic functions of brown fat.[131]

Diet can promote the thermogenic action of brown fat by providing nutrient precursors to noradrenaline, such as phenylalanine, and by providing triggers and potentiators to the activity of noradrenaline, such as caffeine and ephedrine (from the herb ephedra, Chinese Ma Huang). Diet also can interfere with thermogenesis. Excessive consumption of alcohol, saturated fats, caffeine, trans-fatty acids such as are found in all margarines and most commercial vegetable oils, deficiencies of zinc, magnesium and vitamin B-6, and cigarette smoking all interfere with the body's internal conversion of essential fatty acids into the fats necessary for thermogenesis and for general lipid metabolism.[132] (See again the section on thermogenesis in Chapter 2.)

Why Diets Don't Work Part 2

Earlier we outlined the failings of radical and fad diets. Now that the reader has more information it may prove useful to look more closely at some currently popular diet programs. This is intended to help the reader avoid making the mistake of accepting the next "breakthrough" diet. There really are no "new" diets. All diets are variations of original themes discussed here. For convenience, the following brief review begins with the most austere diets and ends with the most luxurious.

Fasting

Undoubtedly one of the quickest ways to lose weight is to go on a complete fast. Under medical supervision, a fasting patient consuming only water might expect to lose about a pound a day, with men losing slightly more. This sounds impressive until it is realized that the weight being lost is up to 30% lean tissue, including tissue from the heart. Probably more disturbing for the individuals involved, in clinical trials of simple fasts, 90% or more of the patients regained all the weight they had lost within two years.

In any case, complete fasts require that one begin in relatively good health. Those with gout or other uric acid problems should avoid fasting. Also excluded are those with liver or kidney problems, those with circulatory diseases, those with anemia and those with nervous disorders. Doctors overseeing fasts will not even allow their patients to take hot baths or showers because of the danger that the patients will faint, so the degree of disruption of normal bodily functions is clearly extreme.[133] Therefore, complete fasts should only be undertaken in the care of a physician under clinical conditions, and even if these conditions are met, total fasts are not recommended.

FRUIT DIETS AND THE PRITIKIN DIET

Quite a number of diet advocates base their diets on the consumption of fruit. One diet in this category is Judy Mazel's *The Beverly Hills Diet*, and another is Harvey and Marilyn Diamond's *Fit for Life* diet. These books are almost identical in their basic claims, with the Diamonds paying attention primarily to the maintenance aspect of diet rather than any quick weight loss program.

The Beverly Hills Diet brings together some quite reasonable points about food combining with some quite unrealistic expectations of what eating only fruit for two weeks will do for your weight. The advice about food combining is a reworking of the classic Hay System, which can be found completely explained in Doris Grant and Jean Joice, *Food Combining for Health*.[134] That book should be consulted for a fuller presentation, but the basic points are these: proteins require an acid medium for digestion in the stomach, whereas starches require an alkaline medium in the small intestine, hence the two should not be eaten together. The claim is that eating a starch after consuming a protein actually results in the reduction of the production of stomach acid despite the continued presence of the incompletely digested protein in the stomach. In the Hay System, fats in small amounts can be eaten with either proteins or carbohydrates, but in the Beverly Hills Diet, fats can be eaten only with carbohydrates.

The heart of the diet is a period of 7 to 10 days during which the dieter eats only fruit, and very little protein is added until the end of the third week. The third through the sixth weeks remain low in protein and low in cereal carbohydrates. Not surprisingly, people do lose weight on the diet, but then the caloric intake for the first two weeks is only about 500 a day.

There are several things wrong with fruit-based diets. First, protein deprivation during a pseudo-famine leads to large loses of both lean tissue and water from the body. The breakdown of lean tissue protein and loss of water depletes the body of electrolytes, especially potassium, and this loss is aggravated by the diarrhea which usually accompanies the consumption of too much fruit. The result is muscular weakness, and, much more uncommonly, respiratory problems, renal (kidney) disorders and cardiac irregularities.

Second, diets high in fruit are high in fructose. A variety of simple sugars are known to be damaging to the liver, and it has already been pointed out that fructose in particular is noted for raising triglyceride levels and for disturbing fat metabolism in the body. Both the Beverly Hills Diet and that offered in *Fit for Life* fortunately separate fruit consumption from the consumption of other foods—*Fit for Life* is even more insistent on this point—and this at least means that these are not mixed simple carbohydrate/fat diets. But such high a consumption of fruit is not healthful and merely panders to the American taste for things sweet.

The Diamonds and Judy Mazel live in a warm climate (Southern California) and recommend a diet suitable only for an area or for seasons during which the main problem of the body is to get rid of excess heat. Those living elsewhere in harsher climates are unlikely to find this fruit diet so attractive. Likewise, take a close look at the skin of anyone who has eaten massive amounts of fruit for a long time—their skin probably will display the dryness and the wrinkles and other signs of aging which characterize the cross-linkage of sugars and proteins after exposure to sun on a diet high in sugars.

Fruit diets are unlikely to be successful for any length of time. The quick weight-loss which accompanies fruit diets will cause the loss of valuable lean tissue and thus initiate the "yo-yo" effect unless the dieter remains on a radical diet plan. The maintenance diet proposed by Judy Mazel and the Diamonds is itself unhealthful, and probably not endurable for anyone living in a cold climate. There is a final flaw in these diets, and that is the radical reduction in the consumption of fats and oils. This point is best discussed in the context of the Pritikin Diet.

The famous Pritikin Diet was established many years ago by Nathan Pritikin. It cuts salt and caffeine, pares sugars and other simple carbohydrates to 100 grams per day, cuts meat consumption to one quarter pound per day, advocates primarily the consumption of carbohydrates, and, most importantly, insists that fats and oils should constitute at best 10% of daily calories, but preferably only 5%. This last, lower figure is difficult to achieve in as much as even most whole grains contain a greater percentage of their calories as fats than this.

There is little doubt that, at least in its early phases, going on the Pritikin Diet has some strong therapeutic benefits for many people. Blood cholesterol levels tend to come down rapidly, as much as 50% of adult-onset diabetes patients become free of dependence upon injected insulin, hypertension is reduced in as little as two weeks, and weight is usually normalized. As a short term therapeutic diet, it is a success.

Nevertheless, there has proved to be a very large downside to the Pritikin program over time. The diet is extraordinarily restrictive and requires considerable time in preparation. It promotes an overdependence upon grains, and this exaggerates problems of gluten intolerance. Gluten is a protein found in many grains, and even in non-sensitive individuals its excessive consumption can cause bloating and intestinal gas, diarrhea, fatigue and mental instability. The insoluble fiber content of many of these grains proves to be too much for most people, and at the levels found in the Pritikin Diet the total fiber content actually drains minerals from the body. Yeast-related problems appear in a significant number of those on the Pritikin Diet. Finally, these problems are not helped by the fact that those on this diet have tended to consume too much fruit and to use too much apple juice and other fruit juice concentrates for sweetening, thus elevating triglyceride levels.

Most of the foregoing criticisms of the Pritikin Diet, it should be pointed out, are those of a former director of nutrition at the main Pritikin Longevity Center in Santa Monica, California.[135] Moreover, the diet is at least marginally deficient in the fats needed to carry fat soluble vitamins to nourish the brain and nerves and to feed the immune system. Indeed, the ingestion of less than 5% of daily calories as fat is associated with cancer, just as is consumption of fats in excess.[136] At its recommended 7% level of calories from fats, the Pritikin Diet is marginal in terms of the fat consumption required for long-term health. (See the discussion of cholesterol and health in the next chapter.)

The moral of this story, then, is all things in moderation. Keep in mind that there are many variations on the theme of radical reduction in calories and of the use of some special component(s) in the diet. So-called Zen Macrobiotic diets (brown rice diets), for instance, fall into this category, and a number of people have died on such diets from malnutrition. Although one is unlikely to perish from simple malnutrition on the Pritikin Diet, several studies, both in the U.S. and in Europe, of those on similar extremely low fat diets have shown disturbing increases in mortality rates from accidents, acts of violence and suicides. The most likely explanation is damage to the central and peripheral nervous systems and/or inadequate production of brain chemicals due to inadequate fats in the diet.

Liquid Diets and Diet Powders

There are now so many of these that it is impossible to describe more than a small number. Most of these diets are versions of high protein/low fat/low carbohydrate diets. Many are neither particularly good nor particularly bad in themselves, just expensive. The first point to consider is that such diets become unsafe if used to exclude too many calories. Consuming fewer than 800 calories a day without adequate supervision can lead to severe illness or even death by starvation. This may seem odd to those attempting to lose weight, but it actually happens and must not be discounted.

Liquid protein diets unalloyed with either fats or carbohydrates, once a rage, are now thankfully much rarer, for they posed serious health hazards.[137] Protein diets of these sorts do little good unless the protein is of high quality and unless there are adequate vitamins and minerals included. This seldom was or is the case. Without small amounts of carbohydrates, low calorie/high protein diets lead to large fluid losses and corresponding losses of electrolytes; they also lead to fatigue.[138] Moreover, the issue of fats again comes up with any diet which increases protein and radically restricts oils and fats. Too much protein unbalanced by fat can lead to a special form of starvation. In pioneer days this was called "rabbit fever" after the fact that a diet made up exclusively of rabbits and other lean wild game caused severe illness. Indeed, some of the current arguments among university anthropologists over whether humans evolved as "hunters" or as "scavengers" revolve around the issue of which of these provided enough fat for a sustainable diet.[139]

Now on the market are various diet powders which are usually added to water and used in place of one or more meals. As with the liquid protein diets, the quality of the protein and the addition of other ingredients is of utmost importance. Nutrients beyond the usual vitamins and minerals are sometimes included, for which see the individual nutrients in Part Three. An insignificant amount of fiber is sometimes added. More commonly, various sweeteners are added to make the drinks palatable. Fructose is a favorite sweetener since it is dubiously thought to not cause fat storage since its ingestion is not immediately linked to the release of insulin, as discussed earlier, but rather causes a delayed blood sugar peak after conversion to glucose by the liver.

The best of these diet powders offer convenience, but few significantly influence the body to burn fat rather than protein or otherwise grossly affect energy metabolism. With their small amounts of fiber, if used for more than one meal a day, such diets are damaging for the simple reason that they interfere with the proper elimination of toxins through the bowels. Likewise, very low calorie/high protein diets do little to train the dieter for life after the diet. Finally, if a given diet moves too far toward dependence upon protein for calories, it then has all the drawbacks of the original and now discredited high protein diets. That is, pure protein diets put stress on the liver and the kidneys, increases uric acid in the blood and thus encourages gout, and ultimately promote the loss of lean tissue if they are too low in calories or are continued for too long a period of time.

The only very low calorie/high protein products which appear to have real effects are those used medically. One such product developed by Dr. Connelly makes use of nutritional signals to direct energy utilization, a process which Connelly terms "partitioning." Such agents "increase oxygen consumption and metabolic carbon dioxide production at the expense of fat storage independent of energy intake."[140]

Dr. Atkins' Diet and Others Like It

High fat diets were used at the turn of the century to treat Type I diabetes, the form that begins in childhood with the destruction of the insulin-producing cells of the pancreas. Since the body can and will produce its own blood sugar from protein in order to feed the brain, there is always some role for insulin in the body regardless of the diet followed. Needless to say, those with juvenile diabetes invariably died young until the discovery of insulin, and no diet could prevent this.

In adult-onset or Type II diabetes, which typically begins fairly late in life and with those already overweight, diet and exercise often can completely control the problem. This and other clues have led a number of researchers to suspect that excess weight gain is related to insulin production either directly or indirectly, as discussed briefly above. Dr. Robert C. Atkins was one of the first to popularize the notion of dieting by bypassing the insulin mechanism through eliminating most carbohydrates from the diet while continuing to consume both proteins and fats. Atkins' Diet is both high in protein *and* high in fat.

As already discussed, high protein, low fat/very low carbohydrate diets have been common for some time, but not with the particular justification that they bypass the insulin mechanism. Generally the justifications have had to do with energy production, or rather the lack of it on these diets. In the Stillman Diet, for instance, it was argued that protein molecules are so large that they use up extra energy as a food for the body. This diet calls for the drinking of at least 8 glasses of water a day, which truly is necessary to remove the waste products of excess protein consumption and from the oxidation of the body's own fats. Very similar is the famous Scarsdale Diet, designed for use for only two weeks at a time. Both strictly limit carbohydrates and, somewhat less strictly, fats. Both do reduce weight in the short term, but such large amounts of protein are extremely hard on the body, as already explained.

In contrast to these, the Dr. Atkins' Diet allows for unlimited amounts of both proteins and fats, but for restricted amounts of carbohydrates according to the theory that a faulty insulin mechanism is the cause of excess weight. Dr. Atkins also includes a long list of supplements with his diets. His two most recent books take aim at his many critics. (See *Dr. Atkins' Health Revolution*, 1989, and *Dr. Atkins' New Diet Revolution*, 1992.) These works provide a great deal of useful information about insulin metabolism, and they provide even more useful medical references.

There is no doubt that for weight loss, the Atkins' Diet works. Fat stores are used for energy, and hunger disappears as the body begins to use ketones, which are fatty acids produced by the liver from fat, as its primary energy source. Those who are overweight often have difficulty in mobilizing fats for energy for exercise or other reasons, so the diet amounts to forcing the body to perform by a different metabolic pathway the metabolism of lipids. As with the Pritikin Diet, followers of the Atkins' Diet routinely discover that insulin production declines, blood pressure declines, and mood swings may disappear. A more limited form of this ketone-based diet is presented by Dr. Calvin Ezrin in *The Endocrine Control Diet* (1990).

The usual criticisms of the Atkins' Diet include warnings of the potential for kidney damage and cardiovascular degeneration. Even the proponent of quite a similar diet program, Dr. Ezrin himself faults Atkins' allowance for unlimited fat consumption on the grounds that this may lead to ketosis, which causes dehydration and to damaging changes in blood chemistry as the blood becomes more acid and calcium is depleted. However, this charge is a bit misplaced since Atkins does *not* restrict *all* carbohydrates. The Atkins' Diet in essence depends upon the fact that the same *catabolic* enzymes are brought into play whether fat comes from the diet or from the body's own stores, and these enzymes can be derailed by the introduction of the *anabolic* enzyme insulin, which must be used to clear excess sugar from the blood. Atkins allows for as much as 60 grams of carbohydrate a day—about one seventh of a pound—divided amongst all three meals. This amount of carbohydrate is roughly the same as that allowed on the best of the very low calorie/high protein diets on the market.

Many in the medical profession simply assert that Atkins is wrong in his diet prescription because he flies in the face of current attitudes toward fat consumption. In as much as Atkins has been able to provide quite considerable clinical data showing that his diet does not increase blood lipid levels, but the reverse, the issue is not simple. Indeed, a number of top bodybuilders in the World Bodybuilding Federation have recently adopted a diet similar to the one Atkins uses (roughly 40% of calories from protein and 60% from fat) in order to cut body fat and build muscle! These individuals are all undertaking extremely hard physical labor, so the diet itself cannot be a source of fatigue, but must in fact supply considerable energy.[141] Therefore, the evidence is that the diet may have a valuable therapeutic role.

Nevertheless, it likely is not advisable as a maintenance diet. Excess protein is damaging to the kidneys and it tends to draw calcium out of the bones.[142] Eskimos eating their native diet of raw meat and blubber may be vigorous in their youth and middle ages, but they seldom live much past the age of 60, and the women begin to show signs of calcium loss (osteoporosis) by the age of 30. Likewise, modern Greenlanders living on a similar diet are vigorous, yet short lived. But cooking the meat actually turns it into a far greater burden on our immune systems during digestion than does eating it raw. Since it is to be doubted that Atkins or anyone else expects modern Americans to live primarily on raw meat, it is hard to believe that the continuous consumption of so much protein over the long term can be a good thing. Moreover, a large amount of dietary fat is often far more dangerous because of what the bacteria do to it in the intestines and because of the dangers of peroxidation within our tissues than for its role in our metabolism proper, and this drawback should be considered when evaluating any diet.[143]

In conclusion, Dr. Atkins' Diet may actually be a good short-term diet for losing weight and for stabilizing insulin levels. As proof of the dangers of the usual American mixed diet of fats and simple carbohydrates, and as an indication of what can be accomplished by abandoning such a diet, it is also useful. Indeed, it is difficult not to conclude that the diet is preferable to the usual mixed diet based upon equal parts of protein, fats and simple carbohydrates—e.g., the burger, white bun, sweet "special" sauce and fries served at fast food restaurants.

However, again it must be stressed that this does not mean that the Dr. Atkins' Diet is the best maintenance diet over the long haul. Both the Dr. Atkins' Diet and the Pritikin Diet, albeit from opposite extremes, primarily offer therapeutic intervention into the body's hormonal mechanism for controlling sugar and lipid metabolism. Chapter Four provides an example of a more realistic maintenance diet.

The Barry Sears Diet

A good maintenance diet should contain some fat, and it is very unlikely that the 10-20% figure commonly suggested by dieting gurus is the correct one. Research has shown that reduced calorie diets, whether high in carbohydrates or high in fat — yes, fat! — lead to very similar levels of weight loss. The same point can be made regarding longevity diets. Reducing the fat content in the diet has *not* proven to be the important variable; only reducing total calories has made a difference in longevity. Even the standard claim that eating fat leads to a higher intake of calories seems dubious. When normal-weight healthy men were tested under clinical conditions, it was found that a high fat diet did *not* increase calorie intake in comparison with low- and medium-fat diets as long as the caloric density of the foods remained similar. (Protein intake was 12% of calories.) This means that fats eaten as part of a diet containing a reasonable amount of fiber do not increase the intake of calories — as opposed to fats eaten in calorie-dense forms, such as pastries, fast foods or bon bons.

Indeed, if the fat content of the diet is too low, this may actually have a negative impact upon the ultimate calorie-burning result of exercise. Individuals who metabolize fat preferentially for energy (those who are high fat oxidizers) benefit more from exercise as a means of losing or maintaining weight than those who burn primarily carbohydrates. The reason for this is simple: high fat oxidizers spare glycogen stores (the limited carbohydrates stored in our bodies) as they burn fat for fuel; after the exercise is over, the high fat oxidizers are not driven to eat excessively to restore the glycogen to the body. Low fat oxidizers, however, must eat to replenish this necessary balance of body carbohydrate. Since the *relative* ability of the overweight to access their own fat stores is usually less (you wear it because you don't burn it), this suggests that a maintenance diet should contain a moderate amount of fat. A problem for dieters is that although they have considerable fat of their own to burn for fuel, their glycogen stores are already only 50% to even as low as 20% of what these should be. Thus dieters often find themselves forced to eat after exercise even though they may be burning fat for fuel.

This brings us to Barry Sears and *The Zone*. Sears advocates a diet which consists of 30% protein, 30% fat and 40% carbohydrate divided into small meals throughout the day. The aim of the diet is to maintain very even levels of insulin and blood sugar, something discussed above under the heading of grazing versus gorging. Sears also claims that the high protein content of his diet releases the hormone glucagon, which is the hormone which opposes many of the actions of insulin. A few readers may notice that Sears has taken some points made originally in Heller and Heller in *The Carbohydrate Addict's Diet* and pushed these very far.

The chief argument is that about 25% of Americans naturally are resistant to the effects of insulin and therefore require more and more of it to maintain the balance of sugar in the blood if they eat carbohydrates. High insulin levels prevent fat from being burned and force it into storage. Those who are insulin resistant, therefore, are likely to have problems with a diet high in carbohydrates. For instance, if you find that eating a normal breakfast containing plenty of carbohydrates actually makes you tired and hungry, but that eating nothing or eating mainly protein for breakfast keeps you wide awake, then you may be insulin resistant. Sears maintains that an additional 50% of the population may develop insulin resistance if they follow a diet high in carbohydrates, such as that prescribed by most medical authorities.

In terms of active weight loss, these issues have already been discussed. Therapeutic diets typically restrict *either* carbohydrates *or* fats. If fats are restricted, then the diet will tend towards an increased protein content. Most dieted will find that in the early stages, this high intake of protein will reactivate the thyroid and make life easier. There is plenty of clinical evidence to the effect that high protein snacks reduce calorie intake more than do snacks of carbohydrate, fat or alcohol for overweight individuals accustomed to the usual American mixed diet. And increasing protein intake to 25% of calories clinically has been demonstrated to increase both weight loss (by 75%) and fat loss (by 57%) more than was found on a protein intake of 12%. However, there is nothing magical about the 30/30/40 ratio proposed by Barry Sears and this amount of protein may prove detrimental in a maintenance diet. As pointed out previously, if sugars and refined carbohydrates are avoided, and if half of the plate each meal is covered with lightly cooked vegetables (i.e., there is a goodly quantity of fiber, mineral and antioxidants in the diet), then the rest of the diet will tend to take care of itself. It is the fiber and the mineral content of the diet which commonly separates the thin from the fat. As noted in the section on Fiber, overweight individuals typically eat far less fiber than do thin individuals. Likewise, research has shown that even a 32% sugar diet which reliably makes test animals fat does not do so when the diet is enriched with minerals. Finally, individuals eating the Mediterranean diet, which is typically 35-40% fats, only 10%

protein and 50-55% carbohydrates, have the best record of longevity in the world. Plus, that diet tastes great! Enough said.[144]

CHAPTER 6

THE CHOLESTEROL CONTROVERSY

> **cholesterol** n. a fatlike material... present in the blood and most tissues, especially nervous tissue. Cholesterol and its esters are important constituents of cell membranes and are precursors of many steroid hormones and bile salts. Western dietary intake is approximately 500-800 mg/day. Cholesterol is synthesized in the body from acetate, mainly in the liver, and blood concentration is normally 150-250 mg/100ml....Elevated blood concentration is often associated with atheroma [arteriosclerosis accompanied by pronounced degenerative changes], of which cholesterol is a major component. Cholesterol is also a constituent of gallstones.[145]

Of all possible health risks, the two with which Americans are most familiar are smoking and cholesterol. The reason that most of us are familiar with cholesterol, aside from its constant presence in the media, is that coronary heart disease remains the leading cause of death in the United States. Almost everyone at one point or another has learned that elevated blood levels of cholesterol may be hazardous to health. Out of a concern for controlling cholesterol levels through dietary means, whole new categories of foods are now being created, such as unassimilable artificial fats for use in mayonnaise, in ice cream and so forth. Similarly, vegetable oils now are used in place of animal fats by major fast food chains for frying purposes, and the list goes on.

The usual rendition of the health hazards of cholesterol runs as follows: Dietary fats, especially animal and other saturated fats, are readily absorbed by the body and/or cause the liver to produce fats known as low density lipoproteins (LDL's) which damage the walls of the major arteries and other blood vessels. Cholesterol then collects at these damaged sites and narrows the vessels until blood cannot pass. In classic coronary artery disease, vessels which supply blood to the heart are blocked, and the heart is starved for nutrients and oxygen. Alternatively, as in the case of many strokes, cholesterol narrows the blood vessels which feed the brain. Eating a diet low in saturated fats and cholesterol lowers the risk of cardiovascular and related diseases.

The problem with this picture is that it does not appear to be entirely true! There are many things which can be done to reduce the risks of heart disease and strokes, but removing fats from the diet is a fairly minor factor. Before delving into what can be done to lower our risks, a brief look at the present state of research on cholesterol and heart disease is in order.

In 1992 one of the most prestigious of all journals devoted to the study of heart and circulatory diseases, *Circulation*, published an article entitled "Health policy on blood cholesterol: Time to change directions." The authors of this article evaluated the best studies on lowering cholesterol through dietary and drug intervention which we have on record and came to these conclusions:[146]

1. In both men and women, low blood cholesterol readings are associated with elevated mortality rates from non-cardiovascular diseases. Readings below 160 in men may actually be associated with slight increases in cardiovascular disease, as are readings above 200.

2. In women, high blood cholesterol levels have no association with deaths from cardiovascular disease.

3. In the major long-term intervention studies, whether these used dietary or drug means for lowering serum cholesterol levels, reduced mortality rates from cardiovascular causes were offset by increased mortality rates from non-cardiovascular causes in those populations not already characterized by heart disease.

It should be pointed out that other similar findings have received considerable airing within the research side of the medical community. For instance, at the November 14, 1991 annual meeting of the American Medical Association, Dr. Peter Wilson reported that the rates of heart attack and of angina have not been lowered over the past decade. Death rates have declined almost entirely because of improved techniques of intervention and treatment, not because of a lowered incidence of attack.[147]T h i s is true despite the steady decline of saturated fats and cholesterol as components of the American diet.

Several recent books and booklets have covered in great depth the failure of the cholesterol hypothesis to account for most heart disease. Among these are *Heart Myths* (Penguin Books, 1991) by Bruce D. Charash, M.D., *HeartFailure* (Touchstone/ Simon and Schuster, 1989) by Thomas J. Moore, and *"The Facts and Myths about Coronary Heart Disease"* by the American Council on Science and Health (September 1989).

The most troubling aspect of the recent turnabout in attitudes toward cholesterol, leaving aside the realization that the American public has remained almost in the dark, is that none of the doubts about the cholesterol hypothesis are new. The same report 30 years ago which led the U.S. Surgeon General to require that all cigarette packages bear warnings of the health risks of smoking also indicated that fat consumption as such was not a health risk. The massive Hammond Report, which surveyed well over 1 million subjects, was presented to the American Medical Association's Annual Meeting on December 4, 1963. The surprise finding in the Hammond Report was that the more times per week that subjects ate fried foods— and keep in mind that in the early 1960's most frying used animal fats— the lower their death rates. This is virtually the same as concluding that the more saturated fats that were eaten, the longer the subjects lived. The Hammond Report was deemed authoritative when it came to the health hazards of cigarette smoking, but completely ignored when it came to the issue of dietary fats. Its very strong epidemiological evidence that dietary fat consumption was not linked to heart disease did not fit the current medical model of that time.

On June 15, 1993 the results of the third National Health and Nutrition Examination Study were released by the National Center for Health Statisitics. These results showed that the average blood cholesterol reading for American adults has declined from 220 mg/dL in 1960-62 to 205 mg/dL for the period

1988-91. Most news accounts have linked this decline in cholesterol readings to the decline in death rates from cardiovascular disease (CVD) over the same 30 year period. Not mentioned in such stories is either the success of modern medical interventive techniques discussed on the previous page or the great increase in the consumption of antioxidant supplements, such as the vitamins C and E, over the last three decades. Also not mentioned is the striking difference in the statistical picture between the U.S. and France. American males have an average cholesterol reading of 209 mg/dL, perhaps lower, and a CVD death rate of 197 per 100,000. French males have a much higher cholesterol average of 230 mg/dL, yet they also have a far lower CVD death rate of only 78 per 100,000. In addition, we should not forget that the French continue to smoke at a rate far above the current American norm.[148]

It will be much easier to understand the nature of the confusion regarding cholesterol if the following points are kept in mind: first, the body itself manufactures two thirds or more of its own cholesterol, and it can do this even from a diet consisting mostly of carbohydrates. Some quite small percentage of the populace is genetically disposed to produce far too much cholesterol, but this fraction does not include the vast majority of us. Second, cholesterol is the base for a great many of the body's key hormones and it is found in all cell membranes. Third, a growing number of researchers now accept that cardiovascular disease may be a subclinical sign of problems involving insulin regulation and/or free radical damage. Finally, in all the major population studies done on cholesterol, it was usually next to impossible to lower blood cholesterol by dietary means unless the subjects also lost excess weight.

This last point is, of course, the key. Obesity, especially if characterized by excess abdominal fat (which often indicates lowered thyroid function) can increase the risk of heart disease by as much as 300%. If we factor in the problems caused by excess weight and add to this the modern American tendency to rely upon canned and frozen foods (which through processing lose almost all of their intrinsic antioxidants and many of the naturally present vitamins and minerals), then it becomes much simpler to explain why cardiovascular disease is such a problem in the United States at the end of the twentieth century.

Does this mean that diet and blood cholesterol levels do not matter? Not at all. As a short term therapeutic diet, the very low fat Pritikin Diet discused earlier has proven quite successful for many individuals. Likewise, cholesterol-lowering regimens using niacin, oat bran and the like (see Robert E. Kowalski's *The 8-Week Cholesterol Cure*) have their place in therapeutics. Individuals with cholesterol levels above 200 and bad HDL-LDL ratios are faced with elevated health risks.

The trick is to avoid blaming the messenger for the message. If high serum(blood) levels of LDL's in fact represent the body's attempt to compensate for a lack of antioxidants, then lowering cholesterol levels through heroic dietary measures and drug intervention is a false victory. If high cholesterol levels merely mark the presence of cholesterol-containing hormones associated with the body's response to stress, then the real answer is to slow down rather than to starve the body of the building blocks for hormones. Finally, if high LDL cholesterol levels, and especially high tryglyceride levels, are the result of insulin-resistance and a diet high in sucrose, fructose, and refined carbohydrates and low in vitamins and minerals such as chromium, then the permanent solution is to stabilize blood sugar levels. Remember, the Dr. Atkins'Diet (high protein/high fat/low carbohydrate) also is successful as a therapeutic diet.

Nutrients Control Cholesterol
And Heart Disease

Now it should be admitted that conclusions such as those presented in the Hammond Report have not been thoroughly examined by the American medical research community. Only recently have significant new ways of approaching the issue of heart disease been widely entertained. Two of these deserve some attention here. The first is that of excessive iron in the diet, and the second and related question is that of the adequacy of antioxidants in the diet. Let us begin with the role of iron in heart and other diseases.

Iron is very important in human nutrition, and it is perhaps the most widely supplemented mineral in everyday foods. However, as with other minerals, the important thing is to get the right amount. Too much iron in the diets of children, of men and of post-menopausal women has been linked to increases in a wide variety of diseases, and the common practice of "fortifying" American foods with iron has been harshly condemned by a number of leading medical authorities.[149]

Recently, the journal *Circulation* reviewed evidence show-ing that the extremely high risk of heart attacks characteristic of men in eastern Finland reflects not just high blood cholesterol levels, but also very high levels of iron.[150] As the editor of the journal pointed out, the connection is now being made between findings of this type and the dramatic increase in heart disease observed in women following menopause.

The argument being put forward by medical researchers is this: Men, unless they are involved in very heavy physical labor or endurance athletics, tend to readily collect iron in the body since they do not excrete it regularly. After women stop menstru-ating, they, too, begin to collect iron in their tissues. Excess iron is known to interfere with the heart muscle's contractions. However, the primary danger posed by excess iron is free radical damage. Iron acts as a catalyst to oxidative processes, and in excess it promotes the oxidation of LDL's also known as the "bad" lipids or low-density lipoproteins. The damaged LDL's settle into the walls of arteries and narrow them. In careful studies it has been learned the men who had high blood cholesterol levels who also had the highest levels of iron suffered twice the heart attack rate of the normal population. Furthermore, there is some evidence that those most at risk are individuals who are geneti-cally predisposed to store iron.[151]

Not only infectious diseases and heart disease, but also cancer has been linked to the excessive consumption of iron, especially by men. The likely mechanism is the same suggested for heart disease, that is, some sort of free radical damage encouraged by excess iron in the tissues.[152] Still other diseases, such as arthritis, similarly may be caused or at least triggered by high tissue levels of iron.

In brief, most men, especially if sedentary, and post-menopausal women probably should avoid additional sources of iron since this mineral is already added to many foods. However, it remains well established that pre-menopausal women and athletes may require supplemental iron.[153]

The role of antioxidants in preventing heart disease is thus indicated by studies involving iron. However, the usefulness of antioxidants is far more general than that. Vitamin C has long been known to help control oxidation of low-density lipoprotein (LDL) and therefore to help prevent its deposit onto arterial walls (atherosclerosis). Indeed, a UCLA study published in 1992 surveying more than 11,000 subjects showed that an increased intake of Vitamin C was associated with a 50% reduction in death from heart disease and a more than 6 year prolongation of life.

In 1989 Dr. Linus Pauling discovered that a protein formed in the liver from LDL serves as a substitute for vitamin C when the latter's serum levels are low. Adequate levels of vitamin C prevent the deposit of this protein onto artery walls. The implication is that atherosclerosis is essentially a form of scurvy. Subsequently, Dr. Pauling and Dr. Matthias Rath published an article in the *Journal of Orthomolecular Medicine* (1991) which detailed the causative mechanism of cardiovascular disease.[154] Also in 1991, a combination of vitamin C and the amino acid lysine was used to improve heart function and to overcome angina.[155] Lysine serves as a precursor to the synthesis of L-carnitine by the body, and it also serves to bind the very protein which Drs. Pauling and Rath argue leads to the formation of arterial plaques. The use of the combination of lysine and vitamin C offers the theoretical possibility of reversing this build-up, and it has been shown to do so in one case.

The protective effect of nutrients, of course, is not limited to vitamin C. Similar protection has been shown to exist from vitamin E, beta-carotene, copper, magnesium, manganese, zinc and other such vitamins and minerals which either act as antioxidants and cell membrane stabilizers themselves or act as precursors to the body's own enzyme antioxidants, such as super oxide dismutase (SOD).[156]

The "Diseases of Civilizations"

Coronary heart disease, as is true of adult-onset diabetes, extensive tooth decay and many other degenerative afflictions, might rightly be called a disease of civilization.[157] These health problems often take decades to become manifest, and therefore it is easy to overlook their relationship to a diet of refined and nutrient-poor foods. Excessive weight gain, likewise, can take years to become a seemingly permanent part of our lives and a source of concern. Certainly the damage to the body's regulatory mechanisms can take place long before the pounds begin to accumulate. However, there are some highly visible signs of impending health problems which usually are clearly apparent much before we can speak of heart disease or diabetes or even a "weight problem."Perhaps the most significant of these indications of future problems is the health of our teeth, and we should spend a little time in closing to consider just why this should be so.

We Americans suffer so ubiquitously from dental cavities that we seldom realize that not all the world suffers with us. Various brands of toothpaste are advertized nightly on TV, and brushing, flossing and gargling with mouth wash are routinely touted to solve all dental problems. Yet bad teeth follow the adoption of a Western diet, with sugary British and American diets always at the fore. What is not often realized (because it is hidden by the successes of our medical *intervention* in cases of disease, as opposed to our medical *prevention* of disease) is that bad teeth and degenerative diseases are usually found together.

As one classic text puts it regarding coronary artery disease, obesity, diabetes and hyperglyceridemia:

"Dental caries is [sic] intimately associated with the geographic incidence of these 'diseases of civilization.' Doctor Fred L. Losee...has observed a strong geographic correlation between digestive tract cancer and dental decay. As was noted for coronary artery disease, obesity, diabetes, and gout, the ingestion of large quantities of refined carbohydrates is causally related to the carious lesion. It has been emphasized that this type of overnutrition may be a potentiationg factor in a variety of chronic conditions.

A pathological oral finding which has been observed to occur in relation to coronary artery disease is dental calculus (tartar)...it appears that the rate of deposition is positively correlated with the personal and family history of coronary artery disease."[158]

Virtually everyone is aware of the clear relationship between the consumption of sugar and tooth decay. However, the quite surprising finding around the world is that the consumption of sugar cane itself does *not* lead to cavities! Cane workers in South Africa who chewed four stalks of cane a day had better than average teeth.[159] Similarly, in laboratory experiments mixtures of saliva and sugar and saliva and cane juice were tested on teeth which had been removed, but which had no cavities. Weeks later half of the teeth in the sugar had been demineralized, whereas those in the cane juice had not. [160]

This same contrast between refined and raw sugar exists with respect to diabetes. In a province of eastern South Africa known as the Natal, diabetes amongst the cane cutters, who consume large amounts of the raw cane themselves, is virtually unknown, whereas there are very high correlations between the consumption of refined sugar and deaths from diabetes.[161] In another revealing instance, during the 1920's with the construction of the Panama Canal, some five-thousand workers from the Dominican Republic were examined—these were people who had eaten cane since childhood—and no cases of diabetes were found. The wealthy Spanish of the area, who ate refined sugar in large amounts, were extremely prone to diabetes.[162]

Diabetes and obesity in most cases are closely related, so the importance of this example to the dieter is clear. The vitamins, minerals and other unknown factors in the raw cane made the consumption of it in large amounts a non-issue as far as dental and general health were concerned. Nevertheless, as a refined product, sugar is a deadly enemy to both, for it radically disturbs the metabolism of minerals, insulin and lipids.

As we have seen, most of the same processes which lead to excessive weight gain also lead to cardiovascular and similar problems. It should also be pointed out that obesity is linked to fatty deposits in the aorta and coronary arteries even in young adults and children.[163]

Nutrient-rich diets high in fiber, in vitamins and minerals, in special "health" foods (e.g., spirulina, whole grains such as barley and spelt, etc.) and in quality fats are not associated with any of the diseases of civilization. Lifestyles which include moderate exercise, such as 30 minutes of brisk walking three times per week, likewise are not associated with modern degenerative illnesses.

The nutrients discussed in Chapter Two are offered because there is scientific research to the effect that one or more of them can help rebalance the hormonal and other systems which have become unbalanced in those who are overweight.

APPENDIX

Although most people become energized after taking a thermogenic formula, two groups may display uncharacteristic tiredness when using such formulas.

Those suffering from adrenal exhaustion may find they have less energy. This is a standard result of adrenal stimulation in cases of adrenal insufficiency. A few days of quality rest and an adequate diet usually resolves this problem.

If the formula contains liver protecting herbs such as silymarin, it may help heal the liver. However, those who have nervous energy from excessive liver stimulation or unrecognized liver malfunction may find that they slow down for a period of time as the liver heals itself. Chinese herbalism often refers to these conditions as unsupported liver fire or false liver fire flaring. These syndromes of excess liver activity will be reduced as the liver heals.

Nutritional Analysis

FOOD	QUANTITY	CALORIES	PROTEIN (grams)	CARBOHYDRATE (grams)	FAT (grams)
DAIRY					
Butter	1 TB	100			11
Cheddar Cheese	½ cup	226	14	1	19
Cottage Cheese	½ cup	100	14	4	2
Eggs	2	150	12		12
Egg Yolks	2	120	6		10
Ice Cream	1 cup	300	6	29	18
Nonfat Milk	1 qt.	360	36	52	
Swiss Cheese	1 sl.	105	7		8
Yogurt/nonfat	1 cup	120	8	13	4
MEATS/POULTRY/FISH					
Ground Beef	3 oz.	185	24		10
Roast Beef	3 oz.	390	16		36
Steak Lean	3 oz.	220	24		12
Chicken	3 oz.	185	23		9
Duck	3 oz.	370	16		28
Lamb	4 oz.	480	24		12
Pork	3.5 oz.	200	16		21
Ham	4 oz.	340	26		26
Turkey	3.5 oz.	265	27		15
Veal	3 oz.	185	23		9
Cod	3.5 oz.	170	285		5
Halibut	3.5 oz.	182	26		8
Lobster	3 oz.	92	18		1
Swordfish	3 oz.	180	27		6
Salmon	3 oz.	120	17		5
Tuna	3 oz.	170	25		7

FOOD	QTY	CAL	PROTEIN	CARB	FAT

VEGETABLES

FOOD	QTY	CAL	PROTEIN	CARB	FAT
Artichoke	1Lg	25	2	10	
Asparagus	6 SP	18	1	3	
Broccoli	1 cup	45	5	8	
Brussels Sprouts	1 cup	60	6	12	
Cabbage	1 cup	140	1	9	14
Cauliflower	1 cup	30	3	6	
Celery	1 cup	20	1	4	
Corn	1 cup	170	5	41	
Cucumber	1 cup	6		1	
Eggplant	1 cup	30	2	9	
Green Beans	1 cup	25	1	6	
Kidney Beans	1 cup	230	15	42	
Lettuce	¼ head	14	1	2	
Lima Beans	1 cup	140	16	48	
Mushrooms	½ cup	12	2	4	
Navy Beans	1 cup	250	11	37	
Onions	1 cup	80	2	18	
Potatoes (mashed)	1 cup	230	4	28	12
Soy Beans	1 cup	260	22	20	11
Spinach	1 cup	26	3	3	
Squash, Summer	1 cup	35	1	8	
Sweet Potato	1 med.	155	2	36	1
Tomato	1 med.	30	1		6

FRUITS

FOOD	QTY	CAL	PROTEIN	CARB	FAT
Apple	1 med.	70		18	
Apricots	3 med.	55	1	14	
Avocado	1 lg.	370	4	12	36
Banana	1 med.	85	1	23	
Cantaloupe	½ med.	40	1	9	
Grapefruit	½ med.	50	1	14	
Grapes	1 cup	70	1	16	
Olives	10	72	1	3	10

FOOD	QTY	CAL	PROTEIN	CARB	FAT
Orange	1 med.	60	2	16	
Papaya	1 med.	150	2	36	
Peach	1 med.	35	1	10	
Plum	1 med.	30		7	
Raisins	½ cup	230	2	62	
Strawberries	1 cup	54		12	
Watermelon	1 sl.	120	2	29	1

BREAD/CEREAL/GRAINS

Bran flakes	1 cup	117	3	3	2
Bread, Rye	1 sl.	55	2	12	
Bread, Wheat	1 sl.	55	2	11	1
Macaroni	1 cup	155	5	32	1
Noodles	1 cup	200	7	37	2
Oatmeal	1 cup	150	5	26	3
Buckwheat					
Pancakes	4	250	7	28	9
Brown Rice	1 cup	748	15	154	3
Roll, Wheat	1	102	4	20	1
Spaghetti					
w/meat sauce	1 cup	285	13	35	10

NUTS

Almonds	½ cup	425	13	13	38
Cashews	½ cup	281	12	20	32
Unsalted					
Peanut Butter	1/3 cup	284	13	8	24
Natural Peanuts	1/3 cup	290	13	9	25
Roasted Pecans	½ cup	343	5	7	35
Walnuts	½ cup	325	7	8	32

MISC.

Olive, Soy, Safflower,					
Corn Oil	1 TB.		110		12

[1]"Methods for voluntary weight loss and control." NIH Technology Assessment Conference Panel. *Annals Of Internal Medicine* 1165, 11 (*June 1992*) *942-949*.

[2]M.E. Mitchell, "Carnitine Metabolism in Human Subjects I: Normal Metabolism," *American Journal of Clinical Nutrition* 31 (1978) 293-306; I.B. Fritz, "Action of Carnitine on Long-Chain Fatty Acid Oxidation by Liver," *American Journal of Physiology* 197 (1959) 297-304. Fritz, either alone or in conjunction with various co-authors, performed much of the early work on carnitine's roles in metabolism in muscle, heart and liver tissues. A thorough review of the literature on L-carnitine can be found in Brian Leibovitz, *Carnitine: The Vitamin Bt Phenomenon* (New York: Dell Publishing, 1984). On biosynthesis, see p. 29. An expanded and updated version of this book is slated to appear early in 1993, and it no doubt will set the standard for popular literature on this nutrient.

[3]J. Bland, *Octacosanol, Carnitine and other "Accessory" Nutrients* (New Canaan, CT: Keats Publishing, 1982).

[4]P. Hahn. "Serum Carnitine Levels and Hepatic and Adipose Tissue Carnitine Transferases in Obese Mice," *Nutrition Research* 1 (1981) 93-99; A.T. Davis, P.G. Davis and S.D. Phinney, "Plasma and Urinary Carnitine of Obese Subjects on Very Low Calorie Diets," *J Am Coll Nutr* 9 (1990) 261-264.

[5]V. Bettini, *et al.,* "Potentiating effect of L-carnitine on the in-vitro methacholine - induced relaxation of massenteric arteries," in J.R. Shipe, ed., *"Drugs in Competitive Athletics* (Oxford: Blackwell, 1991) 107-113; and discussion by Michael Colgan in *Muscular Development* (May 1992) 74-75.

[6] *Nut. Rep. Int.* 36 (1987) 941. J.W. Daily III and D.S. Sachan, "Choline supplementation alters carnitine homeostasis in humans and guinea pigs," *JNutr* 125 (1995) 1938-1944.

[7]G.R. Katts, *et al.,* "The Short Term Therapeutic Efficacy of Treating Obesity with a Plan of Improved Nutrition and Moderate Caloric Restriction," *Current Therapeutic Research* 51 (1992) 261-274.

[8]Those particularly interested in trying this method of weight loss should read Durk Pearson and Sandy Shaw, *The Life Extension Weight Loss Program.* There are some questionable claims made by Pearson and Shaw, particularly with regard to fructose, but also with regard to GH releasers as well.

[9]One of the best reviews of GH release, and one done by a researcher who is himself published in major scientific journals, is Douglas M. Crist, *Growth Hormone Synergism* (Albuquerque, NM: DMC Health Sciences, 1991).

[10]E.R. Braverman and C.C. Pfeiffer, eds., *The Healing Nutrients Within: Facts, Findings, and New Research on Amino Acids* (New Canaan, CT: Keats

Publishing, 1986). See also the highly negative reviews of the effects of arginine, ornithine and the arginine pyroglutamate/lysine combination found in W. Nathaniel Phillips, *Natural Supplement Review* (Golden, CO: Mile High Publishing, 2nd edition, 1991).

[11] L. Cynober, *et al.*, "Action of ornithine alpha-ketaglutarate on protein metabolism in burn patients," *Nutrition* 3 (1987) 187-91; J. Wernerman, *et al.*, "Ornithine alpha-ketoglutarate improves skeletal muscle protein synthesis as assessed by ribosome analysis and nitrogen balance post-operatively," *Annals of Surgery* 206 (1987) 674-678.

[12] Phillips, *op. cit.*

[13] Ann Louise Gittleman with J. Maxwell Desgrey, *Beyond Pritikin* (Bantam, 1988) 14*ff*, 72 *passim* ; Udo Erasmus, *Fats and Oils* (Alive Books, 1986) 287-290. A wonderfully witty and useful newsletter which deals with issues related to essential fatty acids in the diet and with nutrition at large is published by Clara Felix, P.O. Box 7094, Berkeley, CA 94707. On GLA generally, see *The Felix Letter* 58 (1991) and also numbers 57 and 62.

[14] K.S. Vaddadi and D.F. Horrobin, "Weight Loss Produced by Evening Primrose Oil Administration," *IRCS Medical Science* 7 (1979) 52.

[15] J. Bland, *Intestinal Toxicity and Inner Cleansing* (New Canaan, CT: Keats Publishing, 1987) 12. Jane Heimlich, "What the Food Industry Won't Tell You About Margarine and Other Man-Made Fats," *Health & Healing* 1, 3 (October 1991) 6-7. Many of the harmful effects of trans-fatty acids have been confirmed clearly and repeatedly in animal experiments. Others have been observed clinically in human populations. It is interesting to note that the Indian Ayurvedic system of medicine traditionally considers highly unsaturated oils, such as safflower oil, to be undesirable as frying oils.

[16] T.C. Fantone, *et al.*, "Suppression by prostaglandin E1 of vascular permeability induced by vasoactive inflammatory mediators," *Journal of Immunology* 125 (1980) 2591-2596; D.F. Horrobin, "A new concept of lifestyle-related cardiovascular disease: The importance of interactions between cholesterol, essential fatty acids, prostaglandins E1, and thromboxane A2," *Medical Hypotheses* 6 (1980) 785-800; C.R. Lovell, T.L. Burton and D.F. Horrobin, "Treatment of atopic eczema with Evening Primrose Oil," *Lancet* (January 31, 1981), Letter. Several recent well-documented popular booklets are available on this topic: Alan Donald, *The Fat Dictator Diet* (Chatsworth, CA: Cheryl/ Trisha Publications, 1984); I.M. Johnston and J.R. Johnston, *Flaxseed (Linseed) Oil and the Power of Omega-3: How to Make Nature's Cholesterol Fighters Work for You* (New Canaan, CT: Keats Publishing, 1990); Richard A. Passwater, *Evening Primrose Oil* (New Canaan, CT: Keats Publishing,

1981). H. Keen, "Treatment of diabetic neuropathy with gamma-linolenic acid," *Diabetes Care* 16 (1993) 8-14; G. Jamal, "The use of gamma-linolenic acid," *Diabetes Care* 16 (1993) 8-14; G. Jamal, "The use of gamma-linolenic acid in the prevention and treatment of diabetic neuropathy," *Diabetic Medicine* 11 (1994) 145-149.

[17]Alam Khan *et al.,* "Insulin Potentiating Factor and Chromium Content of Selected Foods and Spices," *Biologic Trace Element Research* 24 (1990) 183-188.

[18]The best readily accessible recent review of all the pertinent data on chromium is Richard A. Passwater, *Chromium Picolinate* (New Canaan, CT: Keats Publishing, 1992). On the virtues of chromium polynicotinate (Chrom-Mate), see Katherine Olin, et. al., "Comparative Retention/Absorption of Chromium (Cr) from Cr Chloride, Cr Nicotinate and Cr Picolinate in a Rat Model," 33rd Annual Meeting of the American College of Nutrition, October 10, 1992. ChromeMate is absorbed and retained roughly 3 times better than is chromium picolinate. However, bioavailability was not assessed.

[19]*Ibid.;* also see the informative discussion in Elson M. Haas, *Staying Healthy with Nutrition* (Berkeley, CA: Celestial Arts, 1992) 187-190.

[20] *Ibid.*

[21] C.E. Heyliger, A.G. Tuihiluni and J.H. McNeil, "Effect of vanadate on elevated blood glucose and depressed cardiac performance of diabetic rats," *Science* 227 (1985) 757-759.

[22]J.Z. Meyerovitch, *et al.,* "Oral administration of vanadate normalizes blood glucose levels in streptozotocin-treated rats," *J Biol Chem* 262 (1987) 6658-6662; D.J. Paulson, *et al.,* "Effects of vanadate on in vivo reactivity to norepinephrine in diabetic rats," *J Pharmacol Exp Therapy* 240 (1987) 529-534.

[23]Au Rahman and K. Zaman reporting in the *Journal of Ethnopharmacology* 26 (1989) 1.

[24]Vivek Shanbhag, "Gymnema Sylvestre: A Vedic Wonder-Drug for Diabetes," *Health World* (January/February 1990) 34ff.

[25] David G. Williams, "Regenerating Cells in the Diabetic Pancreas," *Alternatives* 3, 24 (June 1991) 1-2, which reviews some of the more important studies.

[26] John R. Roeback, Jr., *et.al.,* "Effects of Chromium Supplementation on Serum High-Density Lipoprotein Cholesterol Levels in men Taking Beta-Blockers,"*Annals of Internal Medicine* 115, 12 (December 15, 1991) 917-924, reporting that chromium supplementation raised HDL levels in patients whose levels have been driven artificially and dangerously lower by diuretics and beta-blockers.

[27] Michael Colgan, "Vanadium: The Bottom Line," *Muscular Development* (March 1992) 14 and 168, argues that vanadium in all its forms is toxic in any effective dosage. Evidence shows that vanadium given in the water supply to rats causes extreme diarrhea and death from electrolyte loss. However, these are not the classic symptoms of poisoning. The type of supplementation used may be at fault for these results, i.e., through the water supply. Toxicity in any reasonable dosage has not been reported for vanadyl sulfate in human subjects. In fact, vanadium has enjoyed extensive use in treating a variety of human ailments with few side effects. Dosages of above 20mg. taken for extended periods of time may lead to mild readily reversable gastrointestinal irritation For a complete review, see Henry A. Schroeder, Joseph J. Balssa, *et. al.*, "Abnormal Trace Metals in Man-- Vanadium," *J. Chron. Disease* 16 (1963) 1047-1071 and John H. McNeill, *et. al.*, "Bis (maltolato) oxyvanadium (IV) Is a Potent Insulin Mimic," *J. Med. Chem.* 35(1992) 1489-1491. As noted in the text, some informal studies have suggested that the upper limit of an effective dosage is far below that of toxicity, therefore there is no reason to take anything approaching a dangerous dosage since no further benefits can be expected. Cases of active diabetes may prove to be exceptions to this. Julian Whitaker is currently conducting clinicals to determine the effectiveness of vanadyl sulfate for both Type I and Type II diabetes.

[28] Leon Chaitow, *Amino Acids in Therapy* (Rochester, VT: Healing Arts Press, 1988) 79-81. For the anorectic properties of wall germander see *International Journal of Crude Drug Research* 27, 4 (December 1989) 201-10

[29] E.C. Opara, et al., "L-glutamine supplementation of a high fat diet reduces body weight and attenuates hyperglycemia and hyperinsulinemia in C57BL/6J mice." *Journal of Nutrition* 126, 1 (1996) 273-279.

[30] Goodman and Gilman's *The Pharmocological Basis of Therapeutics,* 6th edition (Macmillan, 1980) pp. 253 and 653; Pearson and Shaw, *The Life Extension Weight Loss Program* (Doubleday, 1986) 109ff.

[31] On spirulina, see Christopher Hills, ed., *The Secrets of Spirulina: Medical Discoveries of Japanese Doctors,* trans. by Robert Wargo (Boulder Creek, CA: University of the Trees Press, 1980). See nutrient partioning in Ch.5 below.

[32] Pearson and Shaw, *op. cit.,* pp. 109ff; Leon Chaitow, *Amino Acids In Therapy* (Rochester, VT: Healing Arts Press, 1988) 58-61.

[33] Lucien Abenhaim, et al., "Appetite-suppressant drugs and the risk of primary pulmonary hypertension." *The New England Journal of Medicine* 335, 9 (August 29, 1996) 609-16.

[34] Michael Murray and Joseph Pizzorno, *Encyclopedia of Natural Medicine*

(Rocklin, CA: Prima Publishing, 1991) 53-4, 56, 167, and elsewhere covers the various benefits of these and includes elaborate references. Chapter 5, Digestion (pp. 50-56) is well worth consulting on the general issues. More specific and technical information, especially on Wobenzyme, can be found in the following articles: I. Innerfield, *Enzymes in Clinical Medicine* (New York: McGraw Hill, 1960).I. Horger, "Enzyme Therapy in Multiple Rheumatic Diseases," *Therapiewoche* 33, pp. 3948-57; C. Steffen, *et.al.*, Enzyme Therapy in Comparison with Immune Complex Determinations in Chronic Polyarteritis," *Rheumatologie* 44 (1985) 51-6; K. Ransberger,"Enzyme Treatment of Immune Complex Disease," *Arthritis Rheuma* 8 (1986) 16-19; G. Stauder,*et. al.*, "The Use of Hydrolytic Enzymes as Adjuvant Therapy in AIDS/ARC/LAS Patients,"*Biomedical Pharmacotherapeutics* 42 (1988) 31-34.D.H. Dean and R.N. Hiramoto, "Weight loss during pancreatin feeding of rats," *Nutrition Reports International* 29 (1984) 167-72.

[35] M. Leuti and M. Vignali, "Influence of bromelain on penetration of antibiotics in uterus, salpinx and ovary," *Drugs Under Exp. Clin. Res.* 4 (1978) 45-48.

[36] S. Sugiyama, M. Kitazawa, T. Ozawa, K. Suzuki and Y. Izawa, "Antioxidative effect of coenzyme Q_{10}," *Experientia* 36 (1980) 1002-1003; K. Folkers, "Relationships between coenzyme Q and vitamin E," *American Journal of Clinical Nutrition* 27 (1974) 1026-1034. Folkers, a doctor at the University of Texas, has done much of the research on this proto-vitamin.

[37] Emile G. Bliznakov and Gerald L. Hunt, *The Miracle Nutrient Coenzyme CoQ_{10}* (New York: Bantam Books, 1986) 150-154 citing the Belgian studies of Dr. Luc Van Gaal and his colleagues.

[38] K. Folkers, *et al.*, eds. *Biomedical and Clinical Aspects of CoEnzyme Q* (London: Elsevier Science Publishers, 1991) 513-520.

[39] See the general review in Brian Leibovitz, "CoEnzyme Q," *Nutrition & Fitness* X, 3 & 4 (1991) 47-48.

[40] P. Paranjpe, P. Patki and B. Patwardhan, "Ayurvedic treatment of obesity: a randomized double-blind, placebo-controlled clinical trial." *Journal of Ethnopharmacology* 29, 1 (1990) 1-11.

[41] A.C. Sullivan and J. Triscari, "Metabolic regulation as a control for lipid disorders. I. Influence of (-)-hydroxycitrate on experimentally induced obesity in the rodent," *American Journal of Clinical Nutrition* 30, 5 (May 1977) 767-776; A.C. Sullivan, J. Triscari and H.E. Spiegel, "Metabolic regulation as a control for lipid disorders. II. Influence of (-)-hydroxycitrate on genetically and experimentially induced hypertriglycerdemia in the rat," *American Journal of Clinical Nutrition* 30, 5 (May 1977) 777-784; R. Nageswara Rao and K.K

Sakariah,"Lipid-lowering and antiobesity effect of (-) hydroxycitric acid," *Nutrition Research* 8, 2 (1988) 209-212; Theo A. Berkhout, et. al., "The effect of (-)-hydroxycitrate on the activity of the low-density-lipoprotein receptor and 3-hydroxy-3-methylglutaryl-CoA reductase levels in the human hepatoma cell line Hep G2," *Biochemical Journal* 272,1 (1990) 181-186.

[42] E. Racz-Kotilla, G. Racz and A. Solomon, "The action of *Taraxacum officinale* extracts on the body weight and diuresis of laboratory animals," *Planta Medica* 26 (1974) 212-217.

[43]Anonymous, "Choline: a conditionally essential nutrient for humans," *Nutr. Review* 50 (1992) 112-114. J.W. Daily III and D.S. Sachan, "Choline supplementation alters carnitine homeostasis in humans and guinea pigs," *JNutr* 125 (1995) 1938-1944.

[44]Jeffrey Bland, *Choline, Lecithin, Inositol and Other "Accessory" Nutrients* (New Canaan, CT: Keats Publishing, 1982).

[45]Julian Whitaker, "New Hope on Obesity and Diabetes," *Health and Healing* 2, 11 (October 1992) 4-5, 8.

[46]*Ibid.*,;D.L. Coleman, *et al.*, "Therapeutic effects of dehydroepiandrosterone (DHEA) in diabetic mice," *Diabetes* 31 (1982) 830-833; "Effect of genetic background on the therapeutic effects of dehydroepiandrosterone (DHEA) in diabetes-obesity mutants in aged normal mice," *Diabetes* 33 (1984) 26; "Antiobesity effects of etiocholanolones in diabetes *(db)*, viable yellow (A^{vy}), and normal mice," *Endrocrinology* 117 (1985) 2279-2283.

[47]A.A. Tagliaferro, *et al.*, "The effect of dehydroepiandrosterone (DHEA) on calorie intake, body weight, and resting metabolism," *Federation Proceeding* (abstract 201) 42 (1983) 326; K. Yoshimoto, *et al.*, "Reciprocal effects of epidermal growth factor on key lipogenic enzymes in primary cultures of adult rat hepatocytes. Induction of glucose-6-phosphate dehydrogenase and suppression of malic enzyme and lipogenesis," *J. Biol. Chem.* 258 (1983) 1255-12360.

[48] Usiskin, K.S., et al. Lack of effect of dehydroepiandronesterone in obese men. *Internation Journal of Obesity* 14:456-463, 1990; Morales, A.J., et al. Effects of replacement dose of dehydroepiandronesterone in men and women of advancing age. *Journal of Clinical Endocrinology and Metabolism* 78:1360-1367, 1994; De Pergola, G., et al. Low dehydroepiandronesterone circulating levels in premenopausal obese women with very high body mass index. *Metabolism* 40:187-190,1991; Casson, P., et al. Replacement of DHEA enhances T-lymphocyte insulin binding in postmenopausal women. *Fertil Steril* 63:1027-1031, 1995; Bates, C.W., et al. DHEA attenuates study-induced declines in insulin sensitivity in postmenopausal women. *Ann NY Acad Sci*

774:291-293, 1995; Svec, F., et al. The effect of DHEA given chronically to Zucker rats. *Proc Soc Exp Med* 209:92-97, 1995; Clear, M.P., Shepherd, A., and Zenks, B. Effect of dehydroepiandronesterone on growth in lean and obese Zucker rats. *J Nutr* 114:1242-1251, 1984; Porter, J.R., et al. The effect of discontinuing dehydroepiandronesterone supplementation on Zucker rat food intake and hypothalamic neurotransmitters. *Int J Obes Relat Metab Disord* 19:480-488, 1995; Porter, J.R., and Svec, F. DHEA diminishes fat intake in lean and obese Zucker rats. Poster session, New York Academy of Science's Conference on DHEA (June 18-19, 1995 in Washington, D.C.); Bobyleva, V., et al. Concerning the mechanism of increased thermogenesis in rats treated with dehydroepiandronesterone. *J Bioenerg Biomembr* 25:313-321, 1993; Hans Selye, *Stress without Distress* (J.B. Lippincott Company, 1974).

[49]A complete set of references on DHEA is in Julian Whitaker, "DHEA Reference," supplement to *Health & Healing* (June 1992).

[50]Low levels of DHEA have been found in women as much as 9 years before the development of breast cancer, and many of those with breast cancer have abnormally low levels of DHEA in their blood and urine samples. (1974) 1395-1398.

[51]Simon Y. Mills, *Out of the Earth* (New York: Viking/Penguin Books, 1991) 273-4; G.E. Inglett and S.I. Falkehag, eds., *Dietary Fibers: Chemistry and Nutrition.* (New York: Academic Press, 1979) *passim.*; B. Ershoff, "Antitoxic effects of plant fiber," *American Journal of Clinical Nutrition* 27 (1974) 1395-1398.

[52]Vasant Lad and David Frawley, *The Yoga of Herbs* (Santa Fe, NM: Lotus Press, 1986) 138.

[53]H. Davenport, *Physiology of the Digestive Tract* (Chicago: Year Book Medical Publishers, 4th edition, 1977) 255.

[54]J.W. Anderson and C.A. Bryant, "Dietary fiber, diabetes and obesity," *American Journal of Gastroenterology* 81 (1986) 898-906; A. Leeds and P. Judd, "Dietary Fiber and Weight Management," in *Dietary Fiber: Basic and Clinical Aspects,* G. Vahouney and D. Kritchevsky, eds., (Plenum Press, 1986) 335-342; P. Wilmhurst and Y. Crawley, "The Measurement of Gastric Transit Time in Obese Subjects Using (24) Na and the Effects of Energy Content and Guar Gum on Gastric Emptying and Satiety," *British Journal of Nutrition* 44 (1980) 1.

[55]Julian M. Whitaker, *Reversing Diabetes.* (New York: Warner Books, 1987); D. Jenkins, "Diabetic Glucose Control, Lipids, and Trace Elements on Long Term Guar," *British Medical Journal* (June 7, 1980).

[56]T.M. Wolever, "Relationship between dietary fiber content and composition

in foods and the glycemic index," *American Journal of Clinical Nutrition* 51 (1990) 72-75.

[57]J. Story, "Dietary Fiber and Lipid Metabolism," in G. Spiller and R. Kay, eds., *Medical Aspects of Dietary Fiber* (New York: Plenum Publishing Co., 1980) 137-52; J. Cummings, "Dietary Fiber and Large Bowel Cancer," *Proceedings of the Nutrition Society* 40 (1981) 7-14. M.A.H. Alfieri, et al., "Fiber intake of normal weight, moderately obese and severely obese subjects." *Obesity Research* 3, 6 (1995) 541-546.

[58]J. Bland; *Intestinal Toxicity and Inner Cleansing* (New Canaan, CT: Keats Publishing, 1987) 12.

[59]*American Journal of Clinical Nutrition* (January 1992) 14-21.

[60] Michael Colgan, "Yohimbine: New Fat Fighter," *Muscular Development* (September 1992) 74.

[61]*Ibid.*; C. Kucio, *et al.*, "Does Yohimbine Act as a Slimming Drug?" *Israel Journal of Medical Science* 27 (1991) 550-556.

[62]A.G. Dullo, J. Seydoux and L. Girardier, "Tealine and thermogenesis: Interaction between polyphenols, caffeine and sympathetic activity." *International Journal of Obesity* 20, Suppl. 4 (1996) 71 (abstract 08-178-WA1).

[63] "A Pill that Burns Calories: New Metabolism Boosters," *Longevity* (November 1992) 12.

[64] V.K. Babayan, "Medium-chain triglycerides and structural lipids," *Lipids* 22 (1987) 417-420.

[65] Phillips, *op. cit.*

[66] V.C. Dias, *et al.*, "Effects of medium-chain triglyceride feeding on energy balance in adult humans," *Metabolism* 39 (1990) 887-891.

[67] Lily M. Perry, *Medicinal Plants of East and Southeast Asia: Attributed Properties and Uses* (Cambridge, Mass.: MIT Press, 1980) 175; Y.S. Lewis and S. Neelakantan, "(—)-hydroxycitric acid--the principle acid in the fruits of *Garcinia cambogia* Desr." *Phytochemistry* 4 (1965) 619-625.

[68] A.C. Sullivan and J. Triscari, "Metabolic regulation as a control for lipid disorders. I. Influence of (-)-hydroxycitrate on experimentally induced obesity in the rodent," *American Journal of Clinical Nutrition* 30, 5 (May 1977) 767-776; A.C. Sullivan, J. Triscari and H.E. Spiegel, "Metabolic regulation as a control for lipid disorders. II. Influence of (-)-hydroxycitrate on genetically and experimentially induced hypertriglycerdemia in the rat," *American Journal of Clinical Nutrition* 30, 5 (May 1977) 777-784; R. Nageswara Rao and K.K Sakariah,"Lipid-lowering and antiobesity effect of (-) hydroxycitric acid," *Nutrition Research* 8,2 (1988) 209-212; Theo A. Berkhout, et. al., "The effect of (-)-hydroxycitrate on the activity of the low-density-lipoprotein receptor and

3-hydroxy-3-methylglutaryl-CoA reductase levels in the human hepatoma cell line Hep G2," *Biochemical Journal* 272,1 (1990) 181-186. The LD 50 given by Sullivan and Triscari for oral administration is 4000 mg/Kg, which implies that multi-gram dosages are safe for humans.

[69] P.A. Southorn and G. Powis, "Free Radicals in Medicine I: Chemical Nature and Biologic Reactions," *Mayo Clinic Proceedings* 63 (1988) 381-389 and "Free Radicals in Medicine II: Involvement in Human Disease," 63 (1988) 390-408.

[70] This section draws upon the article "Cleaning House" by David G. William, M.D., in *Alternatives* 4, 12 (July 1992) 97-100.

[71] See, for instance, Sandra Goodman, *Vitamin C: The Master Nutrient* (New Canaan, CT: Keats Publishing, 1991); Mohsen Meydani, "Protective Role of Dietary Vitamin E on Oxidative Stress in Aging," *Age* 15 (1992) 89-93.

[72] K.V. Ingold and G.W. Burton, "Bioavailability on various forms of vitamin E," *Henkel Vitamin E Conference* (1991).

[73] *Martindale: The Extra Pharmacopocia.*

[74] G.D. Foster, T.A. Wadden, F.J. Peter, *et al.,* "A Controlled Comparison of Three Very-Low-Calorie Diets: Effects on Weight, Body Composition, and Symptoms," *American Journal of Clinical Information* 55 (1992) 811-817; see the review of data in Robert Haas, "DHA and PYR: New Fat-Burning Aids for Very-Low-Calorie Diets?" *Muscular Development* (July 1992) 16, 168 and 172.

[75] Stephen Langer and James F. Scheer, *How To Win At Weight Loss* (Thorsons Publishers, 1987) 16-17.

[76] See Elliot D. Abravanel, *Dr. Abravanel's Body Type Program for Health, Fitness and Nutrition*, pp. 300-302; also Goodman and Gilman's *The Pharmacological Basis of Therapeutics, 1397ff.*

[77] C.C. Miller, et al., "Feeding conjugated linoleic acid to animals partially overcomes catabolic responses due to endotoxin injection." *Biochemical and Biophysical Research Communications* 198, 3 (1994) 1107-1112.

[78] K. Deuchi, et al., "Continuous and massive intake of chitosan affects mineral and fat-soluble vitamin status in rats fed on a high-fat diet." *Biosci Biotechnol Biochem* 59, 7 (1995) 1211-6.

[79] K. Kagawa, et al., "Globin digest, acidic protease hydrolysate, inhibits dietary hypertriglceridemia and Val-Val-Tyr-Pro, one of its constituents, possesses most superior effect." *Life Science* 58, 20 (1996) 1745-55; research summary from DMV International.

[80] Michael D. Lemonick, "Is the New Fat-Free Fat Good For You?" *The Natural Way* (May/June 1996) 40-45; *Time* (Jan. 8, 1996) 52-61.

[81] K. Dib, et al., "Effects of sodium saccharine diet on fat cell hypolysis: evidence for increased function of the adenylyl cyclase catalyst." *International Journal of Obesity* 29 (1996) 15-20; M.D. Gold, S.W. Fowkes and W. Dean, "Aspartame: research update (Part 1 & 2)." *Smart Drug News* 4, 1 & 2 (1995); J.E. Blundell and S.M. Green, "Effect of sucrose and sweeteners on appetite and energy intake." *International Journal of Obesity* 20, Suppl. 2 (1996) S12-S17; K.M. Appleton, N.A. King and J.F. Blundell, "The effects of drinks containing artificial sweeteners or sucrose on food intake following exercise," *International Journal of Obesity* 20, Suppl. 4 (1996) 67 (abstract 06-162-WP1).

[82] Karen L. Teff, John Devine and Karl Engelman, "Sweet Taste: effect on dephalic phase insulin release in men." *Physiology & Behavior* 57, 6 (1995) 1089-1095, J.R. Cotton, J.A. Weststrate and J.E. Blundell, "Replacement of dietary fat with sucrose polyester: effects on energy intake and appetite control in nonobese males." *American Journal of Clinical Nutrition* 62, 6 (1996) 891-896.

[83] C.C. Miller, et al., "Feeding conjugated linoleic acid to animals partially overcomes catabolic responses due to endotoxic injection." *Biochemical and Biophysical Research Communications* 198, 3 (1994) 1107-1112.

[84] Kisun N. Lee, et al., "Conjugated linoleic acid and atherosclerosis in rabbits." *Atherosclerosis* 108 (1994) 19-25.

[85] Sou F. Chin, et al., "Conjugated linoleic acid is a growth factor for rats as shown by enhanced weight gain and improved feed efficiency," *Journal of Nutrition* 124 (1994) 2344-2349.

[86] Whitaker, *Reversing Diabetes* (Warner Books, 1987) 89.

[87] *Quarterly Report* (October-December 1990). Other studies using human subjects indicate that B-6 may prevent the formation of bladder and kidney stones. K.N. Pavlou, W.P. Steffee, R.H. Lerman and B.A. Burrows in *Med Sci Sports Exercise* 17 (1985) 466-471; Coleman, "Obesity Genes: Beneficial Effects in Heterozygous Mice," *Science* 203 (1979) 663-665.

[88] D. Halliday, R. Hesp, F.F. Stalley, *et al.,* "Resting Metabolic Rate, Weight, Surface Area, and Body Composition in Obese Women on a Reducing Diet," *International Journal of Obesity* 3 (1979) 1-6.

[89] Ibid.

[90] *Lancet* 304 (1992) 409; J. Mayer and J. Goldberg, "Nutrition News," *Washington Post,* October 1991; M.P. Cleary, "Current Approaches to Weight Loss," *The Nutrition Report* 6, 11 (November 1988).

[91] George F. Cahill, Jr., "Disorders of Carbohydrate Mechanism," in Beeson, McDermott, Wyngaarden, editors, *Cecil Textbook of Medicine,* 15th edition,

(Saunders, 1979) 2091-2094; Joseph Larner, "Insulin and Oral Hypoglycemic Drugs," in A.G. Goodman, L.S. Goodman and A. Gilman, editors, *Goodman and Gilman's The Pharmocological Basis of Therapeutics*, 6th edition (Macmillan, 1980) 1497-1523; P.A. Kern, *et al.*, "The effects of weight loss on the activity and expression of adipose tissue lipoprotein lipase in very obese humans," *New England Journal of Medicine* 322 (1990) 1053. Durk Pearson and Sandy Shaw, *The Life Extension Weight Loss Program* (Doubleday, 1986) 10-11, offering an accessible overview of these issues.

[92] Norman Brown, "Mood Food Debate: Mind Over Munchies," *People* section, *San Francisco Chronicle* (September 3, 1992); Richard J. Wurtman, "The Ultimate Head Waiter: How the Brain Controls Diet," *Technology Review* (July 1984) 42-51.

[93] The effects of television seem to be dose dependent, i.e., the more watched, the worse the effects. See C.A. Raymond, "Biology, culture and dietary changes conspire to increase incidence of obesity," *Journal of the American Medical Association* 256 (1986) 2157-8; W.H. Dietz and S.L. Gortmaker, "Do we fatten our children at the television set?" *Pediatrics* 75 (1985) 807-812.

[94] Elliot D. Abravanel, M.D., *Dr. Abravanel's Body Type Diet and Lifetime Nutrition Plan* (Bantam Books, 1983) and *Dr. Abravanel's Body Type Program for Health, Fitness and Nutrition* (Bantam Books, 1985); Jeffrey Bland, M.D., *Nutraerobics: The Complete Individualized Nutrition and Fitness Program for Life After 30* (Harper & Row, 1983); Deepak Chopra, M.D., *Perfect Health: The Complete Mind/Body Guide* (Harmony Books, 1990).

[95] Pearson and Shaw, pp. 9-10.

[96] Elizabeth M. Whelan, M.D. and Fredrick J. Star, M.D., *The One-Hundred-Percent Natural, Purely Organic, Cholesterol-Free, Megavitamin, Low-Carbohydrate Nutrition Hoax* (Atheneum, 1983) 64-7; Calvin Ezrin, M.D. and Robert E. Kowalski, *The Endocrine Control Diet* (Harper & Row, 1990) 8-12.

[97] Whelan and Star, p. 68; *Nutrition Overview* III, 1 (1988) gives a similar list.

[98] K. Brownell, "Heart Attack Risk? The Yo-Yo Trap," *American Health* (March 1988).

[99] R.J. Garrison and W.P. Castelli, "Weight and Thirty-Year Mortality of Men in the Framingham Study," *Annals of Internal Medicine* 103 (1985) 1006-1009; H.B. Hubert, M. Feinleib, P.M. McNamare, *et al.*, "Obesity as an Independent Risk Factor for Cardiovascular Disease: A 26-Year Follow-Up of Participants in the Framingham Study," *Circulation* 67 (1983) 968-977.

[100] Bruce D. Charash, *Heart Myths* (Penguin Books, 1991); Paul Raeburn, "The

Great Cholesterol Debate," *American Health* (January/February 1990) 79-90. Internationally, the whole issue of cholesterol and heart disease is sometimes referred to as "hysteria" within the American medical profession.

[101] Ezrin and Kowalski, p. 12.

[102] Theodore Berland, "Fast Doesn't Equal Faster," in Hal Higdon, ed., *The Complete Diet Guide for Runners and Other Athletes* (World Publications, 1978) 92.

[103] Scott Connelly, M.D., "Nutrients are the key to building muscle and losing fat naturally" in Scott Connelly, M.D. with Bill Phillips, *MET-Rx Owner's Manual* (Myosystems, 1992). A major book by Dr. Connelly is slated to appear in 1993.

[104] P.M. Suter, *et al.*, "The effects of ethanol on fat storage in healthy subjects," *New England Journal of Medicine* 326 (1992) 983-87; "Alcohol Inhibits Fat-Burning," *San Francisco Chronicle* (August 24, 1992).

[105] Kern, *op. cit.*, note 78 above.

[106] Connelly, *op. cit.*, note 90; Ann Louise Gittleman with J. Maxwell Desgrey, *Beyond Pritikin* (Bantam, 1988) 72; Gary Null, *The Complete Guide to Health and Nutrition* (Delacorte, 1984) 76-78. Pearson and Shaw, *op. cit.*, note 78, pp. 79ff, 318-320, argue that fructose is both safe and desirable. Yet even they admit that they must take additional copper to prevent unwanted increases in blood lipids, that fructose is more apt to raise urate levels than is glucose in the diet, etc. The studies which they cite are usually short-term and do not address the long-term implications that elevated levels of urate (salts of uric acid), pyruvate and other products of the liver imply an increased burden on that organ. For an example of the use of fructose to cause hypertriglycerdemia, see A.C. Sullivan, J. Triscari and H.E. Spiegel, "Metabolic regulation as a control for lipid disorders. II. Influence of (-)-hydroxycitrate on genetically and experimentally induced hypertriglycerdemia in the rat," *American Journal of Clinical Nutrition* 30, 5 (May 1977) 777-784; R. Nageswara Rao and K.K Sakariah, "Lipid-lowering and anti-obesity effect of (-) hydroxycitric acid,' *Nutrition Research* 8, 2 (1988) 209-212; Theo A. Berkhout, et. al., 'The effect of (-)-hydroxycitrate on the activity of the low-density-lipoprotein receptor and 3-hydroxy-3-methylgluataryl-CoA reductase levels in the human hepatoma cell line Hep G2,"*Biochemical Journal* 272,1 (1990) 181-186.

[107] *American Journal of Medicine* 75 (1983) 624. For a long list of other complaints linked to sugar consumption, consult Melvyn Werbach, M.D., *Healing Through Nutrition* (Harper Collins Publishers, 1993) *2, 27-28, 33, 47, 96-97, 109, 138-139, 145, 155, 233-235, 266-270, 276-278, 326-327.*

[108] *American Journal of Clinical Nutrition* (1992); *Muscle and Fitness* (November 1992) 24.

[109] K.E. Powell, et al., "Physical Activity and Chronic Disease," American Journal of Clinical Nutrition 49 (1989) 999-1006; R.S. Paffenbarger, Jr., et al., "Physical activity, all cause mortality and longevity of college alumni," New England Journal of Medicine 314 (1986) 605-613.

[110] Centers for Disease Control, Morbidity and Mortality Weekly Report (January 24, 1992) 33-35.

[111] Physician and Sportsmedicine 19, 11 (1991) 151.

[112] James E. Klinzing, "Carbohydrates, Proteins, Fat" in Higdon, ed., The Complete Diet Guide for Runners and Other Athletes, pp. 44-46, table of body energy sources on p. 52; Julian M. Whitaker, M.D., Reversing Diabetes (Warner Books, 1987) 62-77; J.P. Despres, C. Bouchard, R. Savard, et al., "Level of Physical Fitness and Adipocyte Lypolysis in Humans," Applied Psychology: Respiratory, Environmental, and Exercise Physiology 56 (1984) 1157-1161.

[113] Whitaker, ibid.; Muscle and Fitness (November 1992) 20 reports on the work of Richard Pratley of the University of Maryland, who found that "strength increased 38% and insulin sensitivity increased 33% in middle-aged male subjects during a 12-week strength-training program." For the effects of exercise on the basal metabolic rate, see further H. deVries and D. Gray, "After-effects of Exercise Upon Resting Metabolic Rate," Res. Q. Am. Assoc. Health Phys. Ed. 34 (1963) 314-321; G.L. Dohm, H.A. Barakat, E.B. Tapsott and G.R. Beecher, "Changes in Body Fat and Lypogenic Enzyme Activities in Rats After Termination of Exercise Training," Proceedings of the Society for Experimental Biology and Medicine 155 (1977) 157-9.

[114] Interview given to James F. Scheer in Stephen Langer with James F. Scheer, How to Win at Weight Loss (Thorsons Publishers, 1987) 128.

[115] J.W. Anderson and C.A. Bryant, "Dietary fiber: diabetes and obesity," American Journal of Gastroenterology 81 (1986) 898-906; A. Leeds and P. Judd, "Dietary Fiber and Weight Management," in Dietary Fiber: Basic and Clinical Aspects, G. Vahouney and D. Kritchevsky, eds. (Plenum Press, 1986) 335-342; P. Wilmhurst and Y. Crawley, "The Measurement of Gastric Transit Time in Obese Subjects Using (24) Na and the Effects of Energy Content and Guar Gum on Gastric Emptying and Satiety," British Journal of Nutrition 44 (1980) 1.

[116] See Whitaker, passim.; D. Jenkins, "Diabetic Glucose Control, Lipids, and Trace Elements on Long Term Guar," British Medical Journal (June 7, 1980).

[117] Julian Whitaker, "New Hope on Obesity and Diabetes" discussing DHEA (dehydroepiandrosterone) in his newsletter Health and Healing II, 11 (October 1992) 4ff.

[118] Connelly, *op. cit.*; quotation from W.G.H. Abbott, et. al., *American Journal of Physiology* 255 (1988) E332-337.

[119] M.A. Ohlson, "Dietary patterns and effect on nutrient intake," *Illinois Medical Journal* CXXII, 5 (November 1962) 461-466.

[120] E. Cheraskin M.D., D.M.D., W.M. Ringsdorf, Jr., D.M.D., and J.W. Clark, D.D.S, editors, *Diet and Disease* (Keats, 1968) 28.

[121] See the elaborate discussion of the work of Himsworth and others found in Whitaker, *Reversing Diabetes*, pp. 27-45.

[122] Connelly, *op. cit;* Maria C. Linder, ed., *Nutritional Biochemistry and Metabolism* (New York, NY: Elsevier, 1991) 294-297.

[123] Ezrin and Kowalski, pp. 34-37. *Harvard Health Letter* (November 1992) 6. A far more elaborate treatment of all these topics can be found in H.M. Katzen and R.J. Mahler, eds., *Diabetes, Obesity and Vascular Disease*, 2 vols. (Halsted, 1978) and T.L. Cleave, *The Saccharine Disease: Conditions Caused by the Taking of Refined Carbohydrates, Such as Sugar and White Flour* (Keats, 1978).

[124] See Dr. Yeshi Donden, *Health Through Balance*, translated by Jeffrey Hopkins (Snow Lion, 1986) 186. Dr. Donden, a Tibetan doctor, was asked specifically what he thought is the most unhealthful aspect of American life. Part of his answer was this: "I think that although your food in general is very good, you tend to put sugar in everything. It is almost as if you use sugar as most people would use salt; you even put it in hot pepper sauces. You have gotten used to so much sugar that you just keep eating more and more and more of it. It will induce cold diseases, such as diabetes, as well as rheumatism; it will also make great problems in old age."

[125] From *The Food Balance Sheet* published by the World Health Organization (1983).

[126] See the section on chromium. Turmeric, along with cinnamon, cloves, bay leaves and a number of other spices and herbs, potentiates the action of insulin.

[127] Stephen Langer with James F. Scheer, *How to Win at Weight Loss* (Thorsons Publishers, 1987) 8ff.

[128] F. Nomura, K. Chinishi, Y. Satomura, *et al.,* "Liver function in moderate obesity — study in 534 moderately obese subjects among 4,613 male company employees," *International Journal of Obesity* 10 (1986) 349-54.

[129] Langer, *op. cit.,* pp. 35ff; also see below the discussion of the Dr. Atkins' Diet.

[130] *Experientia* 44, Supplement (1983) 26-44.

[131] Jean Mayer, *Overweight Causes, Cost and Control* (Prentice Hall, 1968) 157.

[132] Gittleman, *op. cit.,* pp. 35-7. *Linder, op. cit.,* pp. 294-297.

[133] Berland, pp. 89-92.

[134] (Thorsons Publishers, 1987).

[135] See Gittleman, pp. 9-14.

[136] Gittleman, pp. 14ff, and throughout; Udo Erasmus, *Fats and Oils* (Alive Books, 1986) 287-290.

[137] R.R. Michiel, J.S. Sneider, R.A. Dickstein, *et al.,* "Sudden Death in a Patient on a Liquid Protein Diet," *New England Journal of Medicine* 298 (1978) 1005-1007.

[138] See note 144 below.

[139] Robert J. Blumenschine and John A. Cavallo, "Scavenging and Human Evolution," *Scientific American* CCLXVII, 4 (October 1992) 90-96. The popular name "rabbit fever" is not unambiguous; another form of rabbit fever is actually an infection.

[140] See Connelly, *op. cit.*

[141] Mauro DiPasquale, M.D., "Let the Fat be with You: The Ultimate High-Fat Diet," *Muscle Magazine International* (July and September 1992); "High Fat, High Protein, Low Carbohydrate Diet: Part I," *Drugs in Sports* 1, 4 (December 1992) 8-9.

[142] For those already late in life and suffering from some forms of arthritis or other degenerations characterized by the movement of calcium into the soft tissues, however, this diet may again act therapeutically. See the anecdotal information given by Paul Martin, "Primitive Diets" in *The Complete Diet Guide for Runners and Other Athletes,* pp. 170-177.

[143] For a general discussion of the role of fats in the body, see Michael Lesser, *Fat and the Killer Diseases* (Parker House, 1991). Unfortunately, much of the research done in the U.S. on fats has turned out to be of dubious value due to poor precautions to insure that the fats used in animal or even human tests were not already oxidized — rancid — when fed to test subjects. Likewise, most of the laboratory animals used, such as rabbits, do not in nature consume more than 5% of their calories as fats, and therefore are arguably genetically unsuited to give results applicable to humans.

[144] A. Golay, et al., "Similar weight loss with low or high carbohydrate diets." *American Journal of Clinical Nutrition* 63, 2 (1996) 174-8; Richard Weindruch, "Caloric Restriction and Aging." *Scientific American* 274, 1 (1996) 46-52; Natalie Alméras, et al., "Exercise and energy intake: Effect of substrate oxidation." *Physiology & Behavior* 57, 5 (1995) 995-1000; S.D. Poppitt, et al., "Short-term effects of macronutrient preloads on appetite and energy intake in lean and obese women." *International Journal of Obesity* 20, Suppl. 4 (1996) 61 (abstract 03-138-WP1); Beth C. Bock, et al., "Mineral content of the diet

alters sucrose-induced obesity in rats." *Physiology & Behavior* 57, 4 (1995), 659-668.

[145]*The Bantam Medical Dictionary* (1981).

[146] S.B. Hulley, J.M.B. Walsh and T. Newman, "Health policy on blood cholesterol: Time to change directions," *Circulation* 86 (1992) 1026-1029. Similar conclusions can be found in the *British Medical Journal* (July 4, 1992) and in the *Medical Tribune* (September 10, 1992).

[147]*San Francisco Chronicle*, November 15, 1991.

[148] Harold J. Morowitiz, "Hiding in the Hammond Report" in *The Wine of Life* (New York: St.Martins's Press, 1979) 241-245. "It's More Than Just the Wine," in David G. Williams, M.D., *Alternatives* newsletter, 4, 24(June 1993) 3, citing the recent American Heart Association Conference on Disease Epidemiology and Prevention.

[149]J.J. Bullen and E. Griffiths, eds., *Iron and Infection* (John Wiley & Sons, 1987); E.D. Weinburg, "Iron and Susceptibility to Infectious Disease," *Science* 184 (1974) 952 and *passim*.

[150] 86 (1992) 803 and 1036.

[151]Steven Findaly, Doug Podolsky and Joanne Silberner, "Iron and Your Heart," U.S. *News & World Report* (September 21,1992) 61-68.

[152]*Ibid.* ; *New England Journal of Medicine* 16, 319 (1988) 1047-52.

[153]M. Colgan, S. Fielder and L.A. Colgan, "Effects of multi-nutrient supplementation on athletic performance," in F. Katch, ed., *Sport, Health and Nutrtition* (Champaign, Illinois: Human Kinectics, 1986) 59-80.

[154]"Solution to the Puzzle of Human Cardiovascular Disease: Its Primary Cause is Ascorbate Deficiency leading to the Deposition of Lipoprotein(a) and Fibrinogin/Fibrin in the Vascular Wall," *Journal of Orthomolecular Medicine* 6,3&4 (1991) 125-134. See also Richard M. Lin, "Lipoprotein(a) in Heart Disease,"SCIENTIFIC AMERCAN *Medicine* (June 1992).

[155] Linus Pauling, "Case Report: Lysine/Ascorbate-Related Amelioration of Angina Pectoris," *Journal of Orthomolecular Medicine* 6, 3&4 (1991) 144-146. Cf, The N. Eng. J. of Med. 328, 20(May 20, 1993) 1444-1456, 1487-1489.

[156] Bernard Hennig, "Dietary fat and micronutrients: Relationships to atherosclerosis," *Journal of Optimal Nutrition* 1,1 (1992) 21-23 and other articles in the same issue; M. Rath, *Eradicating Heart Disease* (Health Now, 1993).

[157] Brian Inglis, *The Diseases of Civilization* (Granada Publishing, 1981).

[158] Cheraskin, Ringsdorf and Clark, *Diet and Disease*, p.315 citing several studies.

[159] N.M. Lamont, "Effect of vitamin C supplementation on black mineworkers," *SA Med. Journal* 50 (1976) 198 and discussed in Rudolph Ballentine, *Diet & Nutrition* (1978) 58.

[160] Ballentine, *ibid.*

[161] Ibid.

[162] T.L. Cleave, *The Saccharine Disease* (Keats Publishing, 1975) 89.

[163] G.S. Berenson, et.al., "Atherosclerosis of the aorta and coronary arteries and cardiovascular risk factors in persons aged 6 to 30 years and studied necropsy (The Bogalusa Heart Study)," *American Journal of Cardiology* 70(October1, 1992) 851-8.

About The Author

Dallas Clouatre, Ph.D. is a researcher, writer, and consultant to major nutritional and cosmetic firms located in the United States and in Asia. He has taught at the University of California, Berkeley and at other institutions. His published articles have appeared in academic journals. He has spent many years in the extensive study of both Western and Asian healing traditions.